Praise for
Your Anxiety Is Giving Me Anxiety

"In *Your Anxiety Gives Me Anxiety*, the title itself reflects that once we are in a physical form, the vibration of anxiety naturally comes into existence. This book narrates how what we are born into can be shifted into something powerful. The true meaning of anxiety is beautifully explained within these pages. Elizabeth April speaks through her own experiences and her vibrational connections to Earth and beyond, offering guidance to help every creation in existence.

May the energies of this book release your anxiety with just a single tap and read."

—Renuka Gupta, PhD, psychotherapist

"Elizabeth April is one of the most unique voices on social media, both grounded and visionary (pun intended). In *Your Anxiety is Giving Me Anxiety*, she has her finger firmly on the pulse of what's happening in our world, blending her gifts of perception with deep compassion. With clarity and insight, she guides us through the maze of modern anxieties, not just the social and intellectual struggles we all face, but the energetic and spiritual layers beneath them. This book offers both validation and direction, helping us navigate the turbulence of our times with wisdom, humor, and hope."

—Kaitlin Parsons, advanced practice registered nurse and psychiatric mental health nurse practitioner

"Finally, a book that bridges spirituality and mental health in a way that feels practical and deeply supportive. Elizabeth April delivers wisdom and tools that bring comfort and clarity and empower readers to face anxiety with resilience. What sets this book apart is how it integrates spiritual insight with a deep understanding of the mind and human experience—a combination I have not seen before. More than coping strategies, it's a complete guide for transformation, offering fresh perspectives and actionable guidance. This is truly a resource unlike any other, inspiring peace, balance, and lasting inner calm for anyone navigating anxiety."

—Teresa Oporto, licensed psychiatric technician, associate professional clinical counselor, and integrative health coach

YOUR **ANXIETY** IS GIVING ME **ANXIETY**

Also by Elizabeth April

You're Not Dying, You're Just Waking Up

YOUR ANXIETY IS GIVING ME ANXIETY

A Survival Guide for Thriving in a High-Stress World

ELIZABETH APRIL

BenBella Books, Inc.
Dallas, TX

This book is for informational purposes only. It is not intended to serve as a substitute for professional medical advice. The author and publisher specifically disclaim any and all liability arising directly or indirectly from the use of any information contained in this book. A health care professional should be consulted regarding your specific medical situation. Any product mentioned in this book does not imply endorsement of that product by the author or publisher.

Your Anxiety Is Giving Me Anxiety copyright © 2026 by Elizabeth April

All rights reserved. Except in the case of brief quotations embodied in critical articles or reviews, no part of this book may be used or reproduced, stored, transmitted, or used in any manner whatsoever, including for training artificial intelligence (AI) technologies or for automated text and data mining, without prior written permission from the publisher.

BenBella Books, Inc.
8080 N. Central Expressway
Suite 1700
Dallas, TX 75206
benbellabooks.com
Send feedback to feedback@benbellabooks.com

BenBella is a federally registered trademark.

Printed in the United States of America
10 9 8 7 6 5 4 3 2 1

Library of Congress Control Number: 2025031875
ISBN 9781637747636 (trade paperback)
ISBN 9781637747643 (electronic)

Editing by Claire Schulz
Copyediting by Michael Fedison
Proofreading by Rebecca Maines and Sarah Vostok
Text design and composition by Jordan Koluch
Cover design by Brigid Pearson
Cover image © Adobe Stock / Aleksandra Konoplya (holographic) and elenavolf (paper texture)
Printed by Lake Book Manufacturing

Special discounts for bulk sales are available.
Please contact bulkorders@benbellabooks.com.

To every soul who ever saw me, heard me, and reflected my own curiosities, thank you. Your love and support gave me the courage to speak when silence felt safer.

And to the reader holding these pages: May you find your voice, trust its power, and never be afraid to use it.

This book is for you.

The world needs to hear what only *you* can say.

Contents

Introduction: Welcome, Disclaimer, and My Anxiety

Hey, Anxiety Ally,

You're here because you feel stuck. I get it. I really do. Like me, you've probably tried it all—therapy, self-help books, and maybe even medication. Yet no matter what you do, anxiety keeps showing up and clinging to you like an unwelcome shadow. Trust me when I say this: I've been right there with you. That struggle, that relentless search for relief, is exactly what inspired this book.

It can feel overwhelming, right? Everyone seems to have an opinion about anxiety, what causes it, and how to fix it, but no one seems to have the whole picture. What is anxiety, really? Where does it come from? Why does it seem to be everywhere, affecting so many of us more than ever before? And most importantly, what can we do, practically and realistically, to ease its grip on our lives?

This book is my attempt to answer those questions and give you so much more. It's a deep dive into understanding anxiety, not as some abstract concept but as a very real, very personal experience. As someone who's lived with anxiety for most of my life, I wrote this book for me, for the part of me that was desperate for clarity, for answers, for something that actually worked.

And if what I've discovered along the way can help you, too, then that's the greatest gift of all. Because you're not alone in this, and together, we can take the first steps toward something better, something freer. So let's dive in.

Who Am I, and Why Am I Writing About Anxiety?

Some of you picked up this book because you know who I am, you trust me, and you believe in the value I offer. Others of you have no idea who I am. Maybe this book was gifted to you, maybe it popped up on Amazon during a late-night anxiety search, or maybe you walked past it in a bookstore and felt drawn to it. Whatever the reason, I'm glad you're here. And since we're about to go on this journey together, let me introduce myself.

My name is Elizabeth April. I'm thirty-two while writing this, but I feel much older than that. Ever since I was a kid, I've been able to perceive things that most people can't. Even at a young age, I could feel people's emotions as if they were my own. I could see energy fields around people, communicate with spirits, and experience things that existed beyond the physical. At night, I would leave my body and fly through my house. I didn't know that this wasn't normal for most people. But while my extrasensory abilities gave me a deep connection to the unseen, they also gave me something else—anxiety.

I didn't have the words for it back then, but I can remember moments that were early signs of what I would later come to understand as panic attacks and obsessive thinking—common symptoms of chronic anxiety. For instance, one of my earliest memories of my anxiety is from when I was around six years old. I was obsessed with my Beanie Babies. I had my own names for them, dressed them up, and took them everywhere. One day, I was sitting in the passenger seat of our maroon minivan, enjoying the gentle breeze from outside touching my face. I was holding my favorite little Beanie Baby, a little cat, when suddenly I had a vivid thought: *What if I throw it out the window?* It wasn't just a passing idea; I saw myself doing it. The image flashed through my mind like a memory that hadn't happened yet. I was so horrified that I immediately rolled up the window and held on to my Beanie Baby as tightly as I could, terrified that my own hand would betray me.

At age six, I didn't have the awareness to question why my brain would conjure up that thought, or whether it would actually happen. I just knew I had to grip on to that little cat for dear life. Looking back, I can say that moment was a perfect storm of separation anxiety and intrusive thoughts, but at the time, I didn't know that. My parents didn't know that. And so, like many kids, I just carried on, completely unequipped to understand what was happening inside my own mind. And my parents, though they meant well, couldn't really help me, either.

Side note—when a new concept is introduced, I'll slide in a definition so that we are all on the same page. Keep in mind, these are my own definitions related to the context of this book. If you want to read up on all the definitions, head to the back of the book where I've included a handy glossary for you!

Chronic Anxiety: Persistent, long-term anxiety caused by suppressed emotions, unresolved past trauma, or ongoing emotional overwhelm.

Energy/Vibration/Frequency: The subtle energetic state or "vibe" you emit or resonate with, influenced by thoughts, emotions, and surroundings.

Extrasensory Abilities: The ability to tap into energy or information that exists beyond the physical realm.

Reality: Not a fixed, objective experience but a fluid construct shaped by perception encompassing all that we see and more.

Intuition: The direct knowing that transcends logic and reasoning, acting as a bridge between higher consciousness and the physical mind.

Hyperawareness: An intense sensitivity to subtle changes in your surroundings or emotions, often leading to anxiety.

As I got older, my anxiety evolved. When I was younger, I openly shared what I saw and felt, not realizing that other people didn't experience the world the way I did. But by the time I was ten, I started to recognize that my experiences weren't "normal." Other kids didn't see what I saw. They didn't see energy or leave their bodies at night. So, in an attempt to fit in, I shut it all down. I buried my abilities and disconnected from the part of me that saw beyond this reality.

At first, letting go of the weirdness was a relief; life felt simple. I played sports, made friends, and focused on the physical world. But no matter how hard I tried to be normal, it always felt like there was something . . . missing. That missing feeling grew into restlessness, and by my teenage years, that restlessness turned into full-blown rebellion. I was angry, anxious, and questioning everything. I remember being sixteen and thinking, *If life is just school, debt, marriage, kids, and a nine-to-five until retirement, count me out.* That existence felt like prison, but somehow, everyone else seemed fine with it. So I started looking for answers.

I asked my teachers, my friends' parents, even a priest, "What's the point of all this?" No one seemed to have an answer. Just vague responses and blank stares. That only made my anxiety worse. Until one day, my dad, who had always been open-minded about my experiences, told me he was trained in past life regression and asked if I wanted to try it. At that point, I was willing to try anything. That session changed everything. In just an hour and a half, I saw several of my past lives. In one, I had been a Mayan priest who could leave his body and travel the universe. In another,

I was a Greek "seer" giving messages about the future. I also witnessed a life where I was a healer who died trying to save others. It blew my mind. It also showed me that my deep craving for answers wasn't just some teenage existential crisis. It was my mission.

That realization gave me purpose. I then went off to university, double majoring in political science and communications. I wanted to be a politician or lawyer, someone who I thought could create real change. But before I left home, I took Dad's past life regression notes with me. I started offering regressions to random students in my dorm, asking if they believed in reincarnation. If they were curious, I'd guide them through their past lives. That's how I started seeing clients. Looking back, it was reckless. I had no formal training, just intuition. But it somehow worked. Through these sessions, I started to see patterns in trauma, healing, and life lessons. And in the process, my childhood abilities started coming back. Clairvoyance, mediumship, remote viewing—it all reawakened.

And so did my anxiety.

All of a sudden, I could feel everyone's energy again. It was overwhelming. I had spent years training myself to blend in, but now, I could barely function in public. Crowded spaces felt suffocating. My thoughts became a relentless cycle of overanalysis and hyperawareness. **I had spent my whole life searching for answers, but the more I uncovered, the more anxious I became.** Still, at eighteen, I decided that, instead of resisting my abilities, I was going to embrace them. My curiosities took me in so many new directions: consciousness, quantum physics, and the nature of reality itself.

Over the years, I've explored some of life's biggest

questions. Who are we? Why are we here? And what's the meaning of it all? I can confidently say that, after more than a decade of searching, I know next to nothing. The universe is vast. The mysteries are infinite. But I do know one thing: **We can't evolve if we're trapped in anxious loops inside our minds.**

So, no, I did not go on to become a politician or a lawyer. I'm also not a mental health professional. I learned long ago that real change doesn't happen from inside the system; it happens outside of it. And yes, I have many books to write—books about past lives, quantum physics, and the nature of consciousness. I didn't see this book coming, but I listen to the signs, and right now, this is what's needed in the world. Not only have the ideas in this book helped me to better understand and navigate my own anxious experiences, but working with thousands of clients from all over the world has also given me the validation that this approach, while unconventional, actually works.

If you're here, reading this, it probably means other approaches to managing anxiety haven't worked for you either. Good, because sometimes all we need is a different perspective—one that finally helps us understand why we feel this way. That's how I learned to manage my anxiety. And that's exactly what I hope this book can do for you too.

Why This Book Needed to Be Written

The year 2020 marked a tremendous trauma in human history—a trauma that affected every single person on the planet. As governments around the world mandated antisocial behavior, depression and anxiety surged. Years later, we are still coping with the aftermath of the lockdowns.

Personally, I saw isolation as both a blessing and a curse. Of course, as social beings, we thrive and grow off exposure to others. As empathic beings, however, we can become overwhelmed and distracted by others around us. The events of 2020 forced us out of our current reality, locked us inside, took us away from our nine-to-fives, and brought us back into ourselves. (Besides, there's only so much TikTok scrolling you can do before deciding you're *over it*.) There was a huge spike in people wanting to heal themselves. There was also a huge spike in people experiencing existential crises. With so much extra time, everyone was forced to question their own happiness and purpose here on Earth, just like I did at sixteen. Much of this questioning led people into a spiral of depression and hopelessness, not finding any answers to their questions. But those few who broke through that discomfort did indeed find answers, healed parts, and brought pieces of themselves back together.

Empath / Empathic Being: A highly sensitive individual who absorbs and feels the emotions, energies, and frequencies of others, often beyond the physical realm.

When we become whole again, we begin to live in a world that is very different from the one we grew up in. A world where energy dictates all and material possessions no longer hold their value. When energy becomes the main currency of life, it forces us to rethink *everything*.

Instead of our daily interactions consisting mainly of going to work, being with the kids, paying the bills, mowing the lawn, and waving to neighbors, we become more focused on the interactions *between* the actions. The guilt you may pick up on from the woman in the ice cream aisle of the grocery store, or the lingering anger from an earlier interaction emanating from the man checking you out, or even the stress of the drivers rushing back home after a long day of work. Every time we interact with the world around us, there is so much more going on that we can't see with our eyes. The more self-aware and healed we become, the easier it is to observe these interactions. Basically what I'm getting at is, the more we heal, the more we feel.

Now, that may sound like a great byproduct of the work we've done on ourselves, but if we don't have the tools needed in this new world, then we are left feeling it all without the ability to navigate through it. Therefore: **Once we are freed from the limitations of this physical reality, we somehow step into another prison—a prison of overwhelm, anxiety, and spiral.**

This book needed to be written because times are changing. We cannot observe a nonphysical phenomenon through a physical lens. It's like comparing apples to oranges; it just won't work. We have an entire generation looking for answers and coming up with dead ends. We have desperate parents wanting to help their children but who are left feeling hopeless. We have professionals feeling stuck and limited by the current rhetoric on anxiety. We have old souls unable to progress through to their mission because of crippling doubt and intrusive thoughts.

Soul: An eternal, energetic being of consciousness that exists beyond the physical body, experiencing many lifetimes to evolve, learn, and expand its awareness.

It's time to take back the narrative of anxiety and empower yourself with information so that you can transform this elusive diagnosis into a superpower. Everything in this book is an open dialogue and is intended to spark awareness and change. If you are ready to take this leap with me, then I am ready to lead you into liberation.

A New Approach to Anxiety

Let's be very clear. Again, I am not a therapist, psychologist, or traditionally educated in the field of mental health. I don't have a degree in this field hanging on my wall, nor do I have letters after my name. And yet, I feel no hesitation in writing this book. If anything, not having those credentials is exactly why I needed to write it.

Traditional approaches to anxiety have failed me time and time again. I've learned through my own experience that anxiety cannot simply be cured with pharmaceuticals or even therapy. There's something deeper at play, something far more complex than what the current system is equipped to address. The experts themselves can't seem to agree: Does anxiety come from the nervous system, the brain, genetics, or the environment? Every source offers a different answer, leaving us with more questions than clarity. And while they continue to puzzle it out, rates of anxiety have skyrocketed to levels we've never seen before. Ironically, the sheer amount of information on anxiety is enough to send you straight into an anxious spiral—hence the title of this book.

So I'm taking a different approach. In this book, I'll share what I believe anxiety truly is and where it comes from. More important, I'll present tangible solutions, ones that you can integrate into your everyday life. The language will be simple and accessible. Every now and then, I may use a term like *vibration*; if that's a new concept for you and you want to better understand it, I recommend checking out the sidebars throughout this book, as well as the glossary at the end. I'll also reference some psychological concepts throughout this book, not because I claim to be an expert in psychology, but because I believe in integrating different perspectives. I want to bridge the gap between Western science and Eastern wisdom, bringing together multiple schools of thought so that everyone can find something that resonates. I've always been a believer in balance. I don't subscribe fully to one side or the other; I see both perspectives and recognize that they must coexist as part of the whole. I believe in both holistic healing *and* Western medicine. But when it comes to anxiety, I feel called toward something new, something outside the established system.

And this is where not having formal credentials works in my favor. I am not bound by outdated research or constrained by a particular framework. I have no preconceived notions or agendas. Instead, I've been free to observe this growing phenomenon with an open mind and a curious heart. My only goal in writing this book is to offer real, practical solutions so that we no longer need to rely on a broken system for answers. As I always say, **take what resonates and leave the rest.** If something in these pages feels like the truth to you, then it's meant for you. If it doesn't, that's okay too. My purpose here is not to convince you of anything, but to validate what you already know deep down and to give you the tools to act on it.

At the end of the day, I am simply an anxiety sufferer searching for my own solutions. My hope is that my journey can help liberate others as well. I have no expectations for how this book will fit into your life, and I encourage you to hold the same open intention. Read with an open mind and an open heart; know that you found this book for a reason.

So, let's begin.

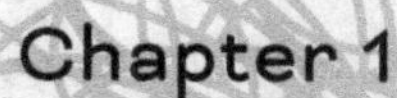

Chapter 1

Decoding Anxiety

Hey Anxiety Ally,

Oh, hey there! Welcome to the club none of us signed up for, but here we are—card-holding members of the Anxiety "Appreciation" Society (membership includes racing hearts, overthinking everything from texts to toast, and the occasional irrational spiral over whether we left the stove on… even though we didn't cook today).

Let's get real. Anxiety is like that overly enthusiastic friend who shows up uninvited to every party, making everything about them. "Oh, you're about to relax? Let me ruin that by telling you about fourteen catastrophic scenarios you didn't even think of." Sound familiar? Yeah, me too.

I see you, I've been you, and I know how exhausting it is to live with a brain that's constantly running around while the rest of you just wants to lie on the couch and chill. So, in this chapter, we're diving deep into this weird, obscure thing called anxiety—*what it really is, why it's there, and how it affects you.*

This isn't just about understanding anxiety. It's about rewriting your story with it. So, buckle up, friend. It's time to turn anxiety into an ally, not the annoying friend who eats all your snacks.

The Spidey-Sense Alert

We are all physical beings inhabiting a physical world. We interact with this world through our five senses: smell, taste, touch, sound, and sight. We live in a fast-paced environment where our conscious awareness is constantly being pulled from one sense to another. Moment to moment, we interact with a world full of tantalizing stimulations from sugar-laced coffee and artificially flavored snacks to emotional TV shows and AI-driven algorithms programmed to keep us engaged. Not to mention, global political fears and a seemingly constant looming financial crisis. **We are locked into this world with our biological systems working in overdrive.**

This sensory onslaught alone seems like an almost unbearable load, but what if I told you there was something else you were interacting with as well? Beyond the five physical senses processing the chaos and busyness of your day, there is another sense that is hard to perceive, but is also working overtime. Some call it "intuition," and others call it "the subconscious," but I'm going to call it your "spidey sense."

Spidey Sense: Your intuitive internal alarm system signaling that something is different or potentially unsafe, triggering anxiety.

Subconscious: The deeper, automatic part of your mind responsible for habitual reactions, memories, and emotional responses beneath conscious awareness.

Conscious Awareness: Fully present attention and intentional recognition of your current physical, emotional, and energetic state.

If you've ever watched a Spider-Man movie, you probably know that his greatest superpower is the intrinsic alert that he gets before something really bad is about to happen. When I first saw him feel and then respond to his spidey sense, I felt it had an uncanny resemblance to my own intuitive connections. I realized that we all have this gift, and yet, few of us know that or notice when it's trying to tell us something. I felt called to use "spidey sense" instead of "intuition" in this book because so many of us have assumptions and existing associations with that term. I want to explain anxiety from an angle you may have never considered before, without any preconceived notions or mental blocks, so we can rewrite the narrative.

I want you to think of your spidey sense as a force that's separate from, but in a way similar to, your other five senses. It is always on, always perceiving, but you probably aren't always listening. We do this often with our other senses as well. For example, when we take a look around, we see the room or physical space in front of us, but we also see our own noses—it's just that our minds filter them out of our mental pictures of our surroundings. Yes, your nose is a constant sight that your subconscious mind chooses not to bring awareness to. Another good example might be the ticking of a clock in your house or the sound of traffic outside. Until something brings awareness to the noise—say, someone comes into your house, and the noise from the street gets louder when they open the door—your subconscious mind chooses not to hear it unless something alerts you to the fact that, yes, indeed, it's always there.

Our spidey sense is a big part of how we respond to the world around us. However, after years of disassociation and distraction, we have lost our awareness of it. In order to fully understand anxiety and then reframe it into something useful, we must deep dive into where this sense originally comes from and how it's getting triggered today.

Where Did the Spidey Sense Come From?

Our intuition, gut feeling, or spidey sense is a survival instinct that led our species to become dominant on this planet. Your anxiety is really a mix of energetic intuition and evolutionary biology.

When our ancient ancestors were out hunting or foraging and they became the prey, their other five senses may not have been strong enough to pick up on the threat. However, that sixth sense, or spidey sense, was there to alert them that something in their environment was different. Think of it as an early warning system picking up on the danger before a person became consciously aware of it.

Now, it's important to know that the spidey sense alert is the initial ping that happens when something is *different*. The alert itself is not negative or positive. However, due to our historic connection with this alert, our biological systems tend to automatically perceive the alert as a signal that something bad is about to happen.

The biggest problem I have had with the current anxiety rhetoric is that nobody else is talking about this alert system. Everyone is so focused on the symptoms after the alarm is ringing that no one has brought significant solutions to the cause of the alarm itself. In no way am I suggesting we need to turn off the spidey sense or try to suppress it—we have enough medications to help us do that. **What I am suggesting is we need to bring our awareness to it and then reprogram our response around it.** It is by no means a quick fix, but I believe it will be the fix you need.

But before we get there, we need to understand how we respond when our spidey sense alert starts ringing. That happens on several levels: emotional, cognitive, neurological, and physical.

The Emotional Response

Although it might seem like the spidey alarm itself is an emotional response, it's not. There is a big difference between the emotional and the intuitive alert systems of anxiety. It's the alert that prompts an emotional response. Then the triggered emotional response can lead to cognitive, neurological, or physical symptoms in turn.

When it comes to anxiety, there are two ways to emotionally process that spidey sense: through excitement or apprehension. Excitement creates an internal flutter of positive possibilities, whereas apprehension creates the complete opposite—fear or worry surrounding potential future possibilities or past experiences.

What is rarely understood is that both of these responses are the same, but expressed in opposite ways. As the saying goes, they are two sides of the same coin. When you think of the word *anxiety*, what do you automatically feel in your body: a good or a bad emotional response? I think most of us immediately sense it as bad. This negative emotional response has been programmed into us as an evolutionary survival skill. In our ancestors' time, whether or not they listened to that feeling determined if they lived or died. It was safer for them to assume that whatever pinged their spidey sense truly was a threat than to wait and see if it was a wolf watching them from behind that tree, or an antelope.

The shift from feeling the initial alert, the "something is different" ping, to the perception of danger or a threat happens extremely fast. In less than a millisecond, our autopilot programming interprets that alert and creates a negative emotional response. **And once the subconscious awareness of an unseen threat has been established, our biological systems start working in overdrive in an attempt to identify the threat in order to solve it or protect ourselves from it.** Again, the alert system itself shouldn't be positive or negative. But these days, our emotional response to the alert system is often working against us, not for us—and that's why we're in this anxious mess.

Autopilot Programming: Refers to the subconscious belief systems, habits, and behaviors that operate without conscious awareness, often shaped by societal conditioning, past experiences, and ancestral influences.

Autopilot System: Your unconscious reaction pattern, where you mentally "check out" of certain experiences because they're familiar, unimportant, or overwhelming.

A big part of this book is addressing the space in between in order to switch the emotional response from fear to awareness. **If we are able to change how our body reacts to this alert by simply perceiving it as positive instead of negative, we can stop our anxiety for good.**

The Cognitive Response

Cognition refers to the mental processes involved in perception, thinking, problem-solving, memory, attention, language, and decision-making. Once we respond to the spidey sense alert with an emotional reaction, our cognition then creates thoughts associated with that emotion.

For example, suppose I light a candle, and as I do, I get an alert since I'm switching the energy. If I respond to that alert with fear, immediately I have the thought, *What if this candle tips over and the whole house catches on fire, and who would be inside and who would call the firefighters, and would anyone get hurt!?* Emotion and cognition are simply *translators* of the same spidey sense alert. The cognitive response may be one of the most important ones to bring awareness to.

In the case of anxiety, cognition plays a key role in the severity and length of an anxious episode. A single thought can spiral into an entire parallel reality where you are seemingly not in control of your own actions or life outcomes. The emotional reaction to these worst-case scenarios makes them feel more real and therefore ends up creating more anxiety. It's a cycle you probably know all too well, and one that seems impossible to escape.

You might think that the cognitive response isn't so important because "thoughts are just thoughts." However, **our minds create our reality.** The mind is one of the most complex and powerful tools we have at our disposal, and no one seems to be using it to its fullest potential—at least not yet, anyway. **Our mental space is our drawing board for manifestation.** We imagine what it is that we want and then we create it in this physical reality. We can blame our minds for our health, relationships, financial status, and even things like our job or weight. Of course, if all of these things are in alignment, then you can go ahead and thank your mind for creating that too! The better we understand our alert system, the more we understand emotions and therefore our minds and our reality. It is that simple and that complex at the same time.

Later in this book, I will share with you the methods that have helped me and my clients overcome this cycle so that you can truly step into self-mastery. But first, let's return to the steps of the anxiety response, because we're not done yet.

The Physical Response

The physical response of anxiety is tangible. Not only is it easy to be aware of our bodily changes during an episode of anxiety, but scientists have been able to study these effects extensively. Rapid heart rate, sweaty palms, nausea, muscle tension, and heavy breathing (sometimes even leading to hyperventilation) are just some of the physiological responses when dealing with anxiety. These symptoms are directly connected to the fight-or-flight response. It's our body's way of preparing for battle. It's technically a protection mechanism that has aided our species for many generations. Nowadays, it seems like the response itself is hindering our evolution, often keeping us paralyzed with anxiety.

The Behavioral and Decision-Making Response

Finally, anxiety ends up influencing our overall behavior. It's the ultimate conclusion to such a complex cycle. Our spidey sense gives us an alert, which then creates an emotional response, leading to a thought, and then a physical response, and then finally when it all becomes too much, we are compelled to do something that will make it all go away. Some people grip the steering wheel when an intrusive thought tells them to drive off a bridge. Others avoid social settings so as not to spark their anxiety, and some act out compulsive behaviors, like tapping on their glass three times to ensure the water in there isn't poisonous.

Rewriting Your Neurological Response

All of this—emotion, cognition, and action—is directed by the physiological and structural layers of the nervous system. This has a lot to do with the firing of neurons in the brain and spinal cord and the creation of new mental pathways. Scientifically, we haven't even begun to scratch the surface of what our neurological systems are capable of and the many complex factors that may affect their function. From my understanding, energy that influences our emotional and mental states can affect and change these neural pathways.

For a long time, it was believed that once your brain has been programmed in one way, it stays that way . . . for life. Like the saying, "You can't teach an old dog new tricks." Recently, however, researchers have started to talk a lot about a concept called neuroplasticity. Essentially, it's the understanding that our brains can be programmed and reprogrammed all throughout our life. What I have observed, however, is that when we choose a behavior repeatedly over a stretch of many years, it creates entrenched neural pathways that are extremely strong. To understand this, imagine walking across a grassy field every day, over the course of years. The path becomes more and more defined as you re-walk it, making it more difficult to change that pathway as you get older. Making a different choice, and carving out a different path, takes work, but it is possible. You need to make different choices to reprogram your brain.

Neural Pathways: Patterns in the brain formed by repeated thoughts, emotions, or behaviors, shaping automatic responses and habits.

In regard to anxiety, our neurological patterns get created at a very young age. Right now, it's common for ten-year-olds to be diagnosed with one or multiple anxiety disorders. Imagine that, at twenty years old, you've already had an entire decade of anxiety created through a negative emotional response. **The more often we feel anxious, the more anxiety we feel.** It's a perpetual self-fulfilling prophecy. As you get older, the list of things you irrationally fear grows. It might move from something like food, for instance, to people, to travel, to your own body, and, eventually, you just decide never to leave the house because it's too overwhelming to even think about going out and interacting. The bad news is that your brain has probably been functioning this way for a while, which means your pathways are pretty set. The good news is that your pathways are rewritable with work!

One way to make a different choice and begin rewriting your neural pathways is to disable the negative emotional association. The next time you notice yourself caught in an anxious response, try giving it a persona to separate yourself from it—like, "Oh, that's just Nervous Nancy overreacting again."

To have the spidey sense dictate how we feel, what we think, how we respond, and even how our brains function is a pretty big deal. **This book marks the end of all that. It marks a new beginning of taking your power back, and rewriting your future.** To be in a constant state of anxiety takes a lot of energy out of us. It's draining, and I don't know about you, but I'm sick and tired of being sick and tired.

And make no mistake—in our world, you cannot escape from things that will trigger your spidey sense alarm. As I've said, I'm not saying we need to suppress it. But we need to become aware of what's setting it off so that we can better manage our responses.

What Triggers the Spidey Sense Alarm?

Anxiety rates are through the roof, and surprisingly, the rates are higher in the most developed countries of the world compared to developing nations. No, we aren't being hunted by a mountain lion as we gather our berries for the winter. No, we aren't worried about accessing clean water to drink. So then why us? What is constantly triggering this alarm when it seems like we have everything society tells us we need?

Funnily enough, we need to observe *time itself* in order to not only understand the origins of our constant anxiety, but also to solve it. The past, the present, and the future are all affecting our anxiety responses. I will briefly explain them here and deeply address them in later chapters with tangible solutions.

The Past

Having a built-in superpower like a spidey sense that alerts you to things beyond your immediate perception is pretty badass. It's an incredible ability, one that can guide you away from danger and toward alignment. But what happens when Spider-Man ignores his own spidey sense? He puts himself at risk. A threat unfolds, leading to emotional or even physical harm.

Now, apply that to real life. Each time we receive an internal warning, whether it's a gut feeling, an intuitive nudge, or an uneasy sensation, and we choose to ignore it, something happens. Maybe we get hurt, betrayed, or find ourselves in a situation we could have avoided. And with each incident, we lose a little more trust in ourselves. We start questioning our instincts and doubting our ability to protect ourselves. Over time, this distrust in our own intuition forces us into survival mode. We suppress the pain, push it aside, and move on.

The problem is, our spidey sense alerts don't stop; they keep ringing. Each ignored warning compounds the last, stacking up unresolved emotions and unprocessed traumas. This cycle begins in childhood and, if left unchecked, follows us into adulthood. Eventually, we find ourselves buried under a lifetime of self-doubt, low self-worth, and emotional baggage we never had the tools to deal with. Think of it like an alarm on your phone. Imagine having one alarm go off every week for the rest of your life. The first time it rings, you don't respond. You move on, but the alarm keeps buzzing faintly in the background. The next week, another alarm sounds and, again, you ignore it. Over time, the alarms pile up, their noise blending together until it becomes an overwhelming, constant hum in the background of your life. Eventually, the noise is so loud that you have no choice but to stop and figure out how to turn them all off.

This is why healing the past is so crucial. You don't have to live with the noise of unresolved pain. You don't have to carry the weight of ignored intuition. **By revisiting the past with the right approach, you can free yourself in the present.** And if you're feeling overwhelmed by the sheer number of alarms ringing in your life right now, don't worry. I have a method to help you navigate through it and regain your trust in yourself. You're not alone in this.

The Present

The world feels like it's ending. AI is advancing at lightning speed, threatening to replace human jobs. Inflation is skyrocketing, making even the simplest grocery run feel like a financial crisis. Your toddler is screaming for more bananas, again, and your inbox is a bottomless pit of people needing something from you. On top of that, your once clean laundry has been sitting in a crumpled heap for a week, silently mocking you, while the dishes multiply like some sort of cruel magic trick. **Welcome to the twenty-first century, where**

burnout is the default setting and overwhelm feels like an unavoidable side effect of simply existing.

When life is coming at you from all angles, it's easy to freeze. You know that feeling—when you're so overloaded that you don't want to do anything at all. You stare at the mountain of tasks, responsibilities, and expectations, and instead of tackling them, you shut down. I get it; I really do. I'm human too. It's no wonder so many of us feel like we're on the verge of a panic attack at any given moment.

But here's what you need to know: There is a way through this. There is a way to quiet the alarms, calm the chaos, and reclaim a sense of peace and stability, even in a world that feels like it's spiraling out of control. We will never be able to fully heal anxiety if we don't start living differently. Healing isn't just about looking inward; it's also about shifting the way we engage with the external world. Later on, I'll introduce you to something I call the oversaturated sponge syndrome, a concept that explains why we feel so overloaded and how we can finally stop absorbing everything around us. I'll share tangible ways to declutter not just your space, but your mind, so you can live a life free from constant overwhelm.

The Future

How does the future affect anxiety? Have you ever wondered what would happen if you accidentally swerved off that bridge? Or what if you get laid off and you can't pay rent? What if a tragic accident happened to you or a family member? I don't know about you, but I've spent way too much of my time worrying about future scenarios that weren't even close to happening. These thoughts are fear of things that have never happened before and most likely won't happen at all, so why is your mind rolling over these possibilities at three o'clock in the morning? It's because our spidey sense is actually a gateway into another realm. Remember, it is our sense beyond our physical five senses. In this way, it is able to perform a lot of cool tricks. Giving us alerts to perceived dangers is just one of its abilities. Tapping into an infinite number of potential realities is another. Once we heal the past and clear out the present, our spidey sense is then free to roam around in the future. This could be a good or not-so-good thing depending on where your vibration is. It gets complex really quickly, but I have the answers you need in order to navigate this space with ease and confidence!

Final Notes

When we look at anxiety purely through its symptoms, it's easy to see how it could infiltrate every aspect of our lives. It clouds our thinking, affects our physical health, and limits our ability to feel joy and presence. But what many people don't realize is that anxiety isn't just a passing feeling; it triggers a full-body response that can have long-term effects. Science is only now beginning to catch up with what so many of us have already experienced firsthand: Chronic anxiety creates a biological chain reaction in the body. Over time this constant state of alert depletes our energy and even rewires our brain, making us more prone to anxiety in the future.

This is why understanding the *cause* of anxiety, rather than just managing its symptoms, is so important. By taking the time, like you are right now, to stop and truly comprehend what anxiety is and why it arises, you are already taking the first step toward deep, lasting healing.

Think about it. Anxiety isn't random. It's triggered by a subconscious alert, something deep within us that senses potential danger, even if we can't consciously perceive or explain it. The problem is, when we don't recognize why we're feeling anxious, our mind rushes to fill in the blanks. We start overanalyzing, and spiraling into worst-case scenarios, magnifying the original feeling far beyond what it was initially signaling. **This is the vicious cycle of anxiety: An unknown trigger sparks fear, we react to that fear, and we become trapped in an endless loop of worry and stress.**

In an attempt to cope, we develop protection mechanisms. Sometimes we suppress the anxiety, numbing it with distractions, avoidance, or even medication. Other times, we try to control everything around us, believing that if we can eliminate external stressors, we can eliminate anxiety itself. But none of these approaches address the root of the issue. Instead, they silence the alarm without ever uncovering what it was trying to warn us about in the first place. And here lies the ultimate paradox: The greatest fear humans have is of the unknown. And yet, the biggest unknown when it comes to anxiety is where it comes from. How ironic is it that the mainstream medical approach to anxiety is to dull the symptoms, making the root cause even more of a mystery? If we don't understand what's triggering our anxiety, how can we ever truly heal it?

Although I will cover strategies to ease anxiety symptoms in this book—because let's be real, relief is important—the real transformation comes from going deeper. **The core of this teaching is not just about coping; it's about reprogramming the initial trigger of anxiety itself.** Instead of endlessly fighting off symptoms, you will learn how to identify, understand, and ultimately heal the subconscious alerts that are causing anxiety in the first place. Once we do that, anxiety stops controlling us, and we take back control of our lives.

Key Chapter Takeaways

- Anxiety is not a malfunction; it's an alert system trying to tell you something.
- The spidey sense analogy: Anxiety is like an intuitive alarm that gets triggered.
- Instead of trying to fight anxiety, learn to listen and decode it.

Key Action Steps

- Start tracking your anxiety: Write down three things that trigger it most often.
- Name your anxiety: Give it a persona to create separation from it ("Oh, that's just Nervous Nancy overreacting again").
- When you feel anxious, pause and ask: What is my spidey sense trying to tell me?

Client Case Study
Jessica: When "Fixing" Anxiety Doesn't Work

Jessica was exhausted, and I don't mean just a little burned out—I mean deeply tired of feeling like anxiety controlled her life. She had done everything the experts told her to do. Therapy, check; medication, check; self-help books, check, check, and check. And yet, nothing seemed to work long term. At best, she got temporary relief, and at worst, she felt numb and disconnected.

When we first started working together, Jessica was skeptical (totally understandable, by the way). "I just don't get it," she told me. "I've tried everything, but my anxiety always finds a way back." That's when I asked her something that made her pause: "What if anxiety *isn't* something to fix? What if it's something to simply *understand*?"

Jessica had spent years fighting anxiety, trying to make it disappear. I explained to her, "Anxiety doesn't want to ruin your life. It wants to tell you something." We began to explore and understand together that Jessica's anxiety wasn't just a normal stress response. It was stuck energy from years of suppression. She had been holding on to so much unresolved emotion, and every time life got overwhelming, her body sounded the alarm.

After months of working together, Jessica said, "It's weird—I still feel anxiety sometimes, but it doesn't terrify me anymore. I'm able to stop and listen instead of react. I get it now." This is what understanding does—it replaces fear with clarity. Instead of avoiding the feelings, she learned to listen and then move through them, to work *with* them, not against them.

By reframing anxiety as an alert system and not an endless spiral to overcome, she retrained her mind to actually process what she was feeling instead of shoving it down. Jessica didn't "beat" anxiety; she reframed it. She was now able to define it, instead of it defining her. Within months, her anxiety stopped running the show. Unlike all the years of temporary relief, this time, it actually stuck. Jessica went from powerless and frustrated to in control and at ease. She didn't just manage anxiety anymore—she understood it—and when you understand something, you stop being afraid of it.

Chapter 2

Anxiety Has a Type

Hey Anxiety Ally,

Welcome back, my fellow overthinker extraordinaire! If you're here, I already know two things about you: Anxiety has made itself a little too comfortable in your life, and you've probably tried more than a few ways to kick it out, only to find it sneaking back in.

Anxiety doesn't just randomly pick its victims—it has a type. It loves people who feel things deeply, the empaths who can sense others' emotions or a shift in the energy of a room before anyone else notices. If you've been through trauma, anxiety holds on to those past experiences like a bad sequel. And kids? Their boundless imaginations make for the perfect anxiety playground. So if you've ever wondered why you seem to have anxiety on speed dial while others stroll through life without a care, you're not imagining things. Anxiety has its reasons for choosing you. But the real question is, why haven't the solutions out there actually worked for you? That's why you're here. That's why I'm here.

This book isn't about giving you another surface-level fix. It's about understanding anxiety at its core, and why it affects certain people more than others. It's about going beyond symptom management and digging into the deep, often subconscious alerts that keep anxiety in the driver's seat. Once we understand where anxiety truly comes from, we can finally do something about it. And trust me, that is where the real healing begins.

The Unseen Victims of Anxiety

What's interesting about anxiety is that it doesn't discriminate. It can and does affect everyone, all genders, races, cultures, and ages across the world. So why is that? It's because anxiety is both an evolutionary alert system and a response to an energetic signal. As we covered in the previous chapter, if you are a human being, your biological systems are wired to respond to unseen threats, and your subconscious is constantly picking up on subtle alert signals from your environment whether you realize it or not. The tricky part is that we usually don't consciously recognize anxiety until we start feeling its physical symptoms. But that spidey sense was firing long before we ever felt our heart start to race or processed what's happening. And again, this is part of being human.

That being said, there are certain groups of individuals who tend to be more affected by anxiety than others. In this chapter, I'll be focusing on the top three most impacted groups, but that doesn't mean anxiety skips over the rest—far from it. If you don't see yourself reflected in these categories, don't assume your anxiety is any less valid. The reality is, anyone can experience debilitating anxiety, even if they don't fit into one of these "high risk" groups. Anxiety is personal. It manifests differently for everyone and is shaped by a unique mix of biology, environment, past experiences, and energetic sensitivity. If I really tried to cover every subgroup that experienced anxiety, we'd be here all day. Instead, I'm going to focus on the groups that are not typically recognized in the mainstream rhetoric but that I've observed time and time again among my own clients, while also recognizing that anxiety doesn't follow rules, labels, or a one-size-fits-all explanation. If you've ever felt overwhelmed, hyperaware, or trapped in cycles of fear, no matter who you are, you are not alone.

Empaths

Being an empath means that a person is a highly sensitive individual. Yes, this may mean that they are more emotional than most, but it doesn't always relate to their emotional state. Sensitivities can come in all shapes and forms. People can be sensitive to the weather, or to too much screen time; they can be sensitive to the news or how the rest of the world views them. **When someone is extra sensitive, their stimulation inputs are on hyperdrive, which means they are prime candidates for an extra amount of anxiety.**

I'm going to take a wild guess here and say that you are

most likely an empath. There are many reasons why I would assume that—one being the fact that you're reading this book right now. You have likely tried alternate solutions to anxiety but haven't found any that really stuck. (That's totally okay, by the way; sometimes the process of elimination helps us to better understand what does work. I hope this book will finally help you conquer anxiety in a sustainable way.)

Empath: A highly sensitive individual who absorbs and feels the emotions, energies, and frequencies of others.

Electromagnetic Frequencies (EMFs): Vibrational energy waves that exist all around us, influencing both our physical and energetic bodies.

Solar Flares: Bursts of electromagnetic energy from the sun, believed to trigger energetic changes and upgrades in your brain and emotional sensitivity.

As you might already know, humans are energy beings. Actually, all life in the universe is simply energy rearranged into different forms. As humans, we each have a soul first, and then we choose to incarnate into a physical form. But if we think about our current existence and what we do all day, our lives consist primarily of physical interactions. We wake up, get out of bed, make coffee, have something to eat, and hop into our car to drive to work. Yes, we live in a physical reality and therefore we interact with it in a physical way. But although we have been led to believe the physical world is all that exists, that is far from the truth. Luckily, with breakthroughs in quantum physics, scientists are starting to study and understand the impact energy has throughout all matter. **And the very nature of our reality is changing.**

We are in the midst of a profound shift, moving from one frequency to another. The energy of this world is evolving, and whether we are aware of it or not, we are evolving with it. This transformation isn't just a philosophical idea; it is a phenomenon that can be measured and studied. One key indicator of this energetic shift is a change in something called the Schumann resonances, often referred to as the "heartbeat of the Earth." This phrase refers to electromagnetic resonances created by lightning strikes between the planet's surface and the ionosphere. You might know that the Earth has a magnetic field that extends from inside our planet out into space, shielding us from solar wind. When lightning (or another electric phenomenon) occurs, it creates a kind of ripple effect in the electromagnetic frequencies in this field around the planet. For centuries, the Schumann resonances remained relatively stable, but in recent years, they have been fluctuating dramatically, signaling an acceleration in planetary energy. At the same time, we are experiencing an increase in solar activity. The sun has entered a phase known as the solar maximum, a cycle in which solar flares and coronal mass ejections (CMEs) become more frequent and intense. These solar flares release massive waves of electromagnetic radiation that travel through space and interact directly with Earth's magnetic field. (You might have noticed that the auroras—northern and southern lights—are becoming more common occurrences now too.) This isn't just cosmic weather. It can damage satellites and disrupt our power grid, and it has tangible effects on all living beings.

Just like the Earth, each human generates an electromagnetic field, a byproduct of our biological and energetic systems. Every thought, emotion, and cell in our body operates within an energetic framework. Our nervous system itself is electrical in nature, which means that external electromagnetic fluctuations, like those from the sun, directly impact us. Beyond the physical, I also believe that every organism has a soul, a guiding force that sustains us beyond our biological makeup. When the frequency of Earth increases due to solar activity and energetic shifts, our own frequency naturally rises in response. This is why I believe so many people today feel heightened sensitivity, emotional intensity, and even unexplained physical symptoms like fatigue, headaches, and restless sleep. **We are being called to align with a new energetic paradigm.**

This shift is not just a subtle background change. It is actively reshaping the way we interact with reality. As our frequency increases, we are being guided away from a purely physical perception of existence and drawn into the realm of the nonphysical. This means our intuition is heightening, our awareness is expanding, and our ability to perceive energy beyond the five senses is awakening, leading to an increased focus on our spidey sense.

I believe this global shift in energy is part of the reason we have such a sharp increase in cases of anxiety. The energy shift is making us more sensitive than ever before. People who have never thought of themselves as empaths or highly sensitive individuals are all of a sudden feeling overwhelmed by simple interactions.

When you are extra sensitive, you begin to bring awareness to all of the energies interacting in and around you. Before, it was easy to make a decision and see the end result of that choice. For instance, you go over to the fridge, you pick up the bottle of water, pour yourself a drink, and then drink it; you are no longer thirsty. Easy-peasy, cause and effect. With this new development of increasing frequency, it isn't as simple as cause and effect anymore. There are hidden energies playing out, before, during, and after the physical interaction. In the water example, your roommate could have poured some water earlier and left emotional remnants on it such as excitement or anticipation. When you go to drink that water, you could be picking up on those energies without even realizing it. You see, when you become more energetically aware, cause and effect is no longer just physical; it becomes more complex due to your awareness around the extra energetic layers. A simple action, like texting a friend, may seem straightforward, but behind it could be emotional energies from the past, or unspoken feelings in the moment. You might feel anxiety that isn't even yours, or receive a cold reply that reflects deeper dynamics unrelated to the text itself. As your frequency rises, you begin to sense the invisible forces influencing your choices, interactions, and outcomes, before, during, and after they happen.

There is a whole world behind and beyond the one we were raised in. And these days, that world is becoming more and more apparent. Just as we have been taught to do maintenance on our physical lives and selves, like taking a shower, paying our bills, and eating a healthy diet, we need to learn to listen and respond to the energetic world—just as much, if not more. As we become more sensitive to these small energetic interactions, our spidey sense alerts are ringing in all directions.

When we begin to pick up on the energies around us, we can also become attuned to the vibrations and energies (and emotions) of other people. For example, let's say you go to the grocery store to grab dinner for the night. As usual, you peruse the aisles to find your go-to meal. You stand in line and have the cashier check you out. Taking out your wallet and paying, you feel an intense sense of sadness. When you look up, you see it in the cashier's eyes. You ask him if he's okay, and he responds with a weak "yeah, I'm fine." Although you verbally heard the response that he was okay, you know he isn't. You feel that he is grieving; you sense that he lost someone who was really close to him, maybe a parent. You feel like he's at work because he needs to be—beyond earning money, his job might help take his mind off things. Your focus is quickly diverted from those feelings and back into the present moment as the credit card reader beeps, prompting you to pay. It all happened so fast and so quietly you forget about the cashier the second you get home . . . but that's when the symptoms start. Your heart rate picks up, you begin to sweat, and your mind is racing. Fears about your work presentation next week are spiraling around; a twisting sensation in your stomach makes you feel nauseous. You sit down to try to focus on your breathing. You have no idea why you feel this way or where it's coming from. You utilize your mindfulness techniques or maybe even your medication to stop the symptoms and start to feel better. When you start feeling better, you don't give the anxious moment a second thought and go to bed.

What many of us don't realize is that every action, reaction, thought, and emotion creates an energetic ripple into our environment. Anxiety often comes up in response to such an energetic alert, signaling that something feels off, wrong, or difficult to perceive consciously. As we become more sensitive to the energy around us, these alerts become more frequent and active.

Empaths, or those who are highly sensitive to energies, are more prone to anxiety because they're constantly processing the world around them on a deeper level. If we don't learn how to manage these energies, even simple moments can start to feel overwhelming and unmanageable. This heightened sensitivity is also why empaths often experience social anxiety. Before heading out for a night with friends, your spidey sense alarm is going off. Your system already knows that being around a large group of people will mean a significant influx of energy. Your mind tries to interpret this warning, often focusing on external fears: *Will I be judged for what I'm wearing? Who's going to be there? How will they perceive me?* But the truth is, your anxiety isn't about the judgments of others; it's about bracing for the energetic overwhelm you're about to experience. **Your system is trying to protect you, even if your mind misinterprets the message.** Later, I'll guide you on how to reprogram these alerts so they align with your own intuitive insights, rather than being overwhelmed by the interactions from your surroundings.

Trauma Survivors

If we're talking about who anxiety affects the most, trauma survivors might just be at the top of the list. But before you think, *Well, I haven't had major trauma, so this doesn't apply to me*, and check out, stay with me for a second. Trauma isn't just about catastrophic events. The term is not reserved for war veterans, abuse survivors, or those who have faced extreme hardship. Trauma comes in many different shapes and sizes. For some, trauma is the obvious stuff—being in and out of the foster care system, growing up with parents who struggled with addiction, or experiencing violence, abuse, or neglect. For others, trauma is quieter, and less visible from the outside. It could be being bullied in childhood, feeling unseen or unheard in your own home, struggling with perfectionism, experiencing repeated rejection, or being forced into roles and expectations that never truly fit you.

A trauma survivor, in simplest terms, is someone who has been through something difficult and made it to the other side. And surviving doesn't mean we're thriving. Just because we move past an event doesn't mean it hasn't left a lasting imprint on our nervous system, our emotions, and the way we interact with the world. And that's the thing about trauma: It's not just about what happened to us; it's about how our body, mind, and energy processed (or didn't process) those experiences.

What defines trauma is not the event itself, but how it was experienced. The same situation can affect two people in completely different ways. One person's worst day could be another person's best day. That's why trauma is so hard to categorize, and why it can't be measured by external standards.

This is also why we can never definitively say which traumas will lead to the most anxiety. They are all equally relevant. The traumas that will impact our anxiety the most, however, are the ones that have gone **unresolved**. When painful experiences aren't fully processed, whether they happened last year or decades ago, they don't just fade away. They linger in our subconscious, shaping our fears, our reactions, and the way we navigate life. **Anxiety, in many ways, is a direct response to unresolved trauma.** It's our nervous system saying, "Something still feels unsafe."

So if you identify with this, then it's time to finally understand how these traumas could be still affecting you, despite your awareness of it.

Suppressed Emotions Leading to Oversaturated Sponge Syndrome

During a traumatic experience, our nervous system often activates the fight, flight, or freeze response, a survival mechanism designed to help us navigate and endure the threat. One way our nervous system protects us is through *dissociation.* By disconnecting from the trauma in the moment, we can focus on surviving and moving forward. In the moment, dissociation serves as a coping tool, allowing us to suppress intense emotions and approach the situation more logically. However, as you may know, dissociation can have significant long-term consequences. Those unresolved emotions don't simply disappear; they accumulate beneath the surface, often resurfacing later with an even greater impact, perpetuating the cycle of trauma and creating a lot of anxiety.

Fight, Flight, or Freeze Response: Your automatic survival reaction when feeling threatened, either fighting, fleeing, or becoming frozen and inactive.

Dissociation: When your conscious awareness disconnects from the present moment, either from your physical body, emotional state, or environment, usually as a protective mechanism.

Oversaturated Sponge Syndrome: Feeling overwhelmed due to absorbing too many emotions, energies, or external inputs, causing exhaustion and anxiety.

This concept was so dominant in my client sessions, I came up with a term describing this problem: the *oversaturated sponge syndrome*. Imagine a dry sponge sitting in your kitchen sink. Now imagine you turn the water on and fill up that sponge. Eventually, it'll get to a point where the sponge is so full of water even just one more drop in will prompt a downpour of drainage. If you haven't already picked up on it, in this metaphor the sponge is you, and the water is energy, emotion, and/or trauma. The more we take on without letting go, the more prone we are to becoming the oversaturated sponge. Here's a little test to see whether or not you are currently in this state.

Quiz: Are You an Oversaturated Sponge?

Instructions: Answer each question with a simple "Yes" or "No." For every "Yes," give yourself 1 point. At the end, tally your score.

1. Do you feel triggered often?
2. Do you feel out of control with your own emotions?
3. Do you feel anxious often?
4. Do you feel fed up with the state of the world?
5. Do you often feel overwhelmed?
6. Do you feel constantly tired regardless of how much sleep you get?
7. Do you have a hard time quieting your mind?
8. Do you feel like no one understands you?

Your Score & Results

0–3 Points: Balanced

Congratulations. It seems like you have a good balance. You've put in some work to release the old energy. Yes, we all have bad days, but for the most part, you are ensuring that you set boundaries and have self-love mechanisms in place to combat them.

4–6 Points: Taking On Water

It's clear that an accumulation of energies is negatively impacting your quality of life. It's time to rearrange some things and focus on you for once!

7–8 Points: Oversaturation Reached

You are the oversaturated sponge and it's time to change that!

As a trauma survivor, you have a lot of experiences under your belt. This makes you a beautifully unique and well-rounded individual. However, this isn't a case of "what doesn't kill you makes you stronger." What you endured may have made you stronger, but it most likely still affects your overall quality of life, especially if you are a chronic anxiety sufferer. Later on, I will go over my techniques, which will help you drain your sponge *and* keep it drained so that you have the capacity to show up presently, without fears, anxieties, or suppressed traumas.

Loss of Self-Worth

A trauma survivor will also experience more anxiety because they are prone to more fears overall. Now, it's easy to say that if you get mugged in a back alley walking alone, you will have a fear of walking alone, or leaving the house, or even meeting strangers because of it. Although it's clear that an experience like that would have a negative impact on you,

I've found that the deeper root of anxiety doesn't come from the past danger itself; it comes from the loss of trust in ourselves that follows.

As I discussed in chapter one, anxiety starts from a spidey sense alert, which usually goes unnoticed, and sometimes something bad does happen. Eventually, when we look back to see the warning signs, we feel disappointed in ourselves for the lack of awareness. Sometimes this disappointment is conscious, but most of the time it's deeply subconscious. The warnings are there, the intuition is present, and yet we just didn't listen.

We are taught to direct our focus to the physical world through our five senses, rather than the energetic world through our spidey sense. When we live our entire lives like this, it begins to wear on us, creating a deep sense of mistrust in our own choices and judgment. The fear of the unknown is not because something bad could happen; it's because we've lost trust in ourselves to listen to the signals. It's not a trust issue with the world; it's a trust issue with yourself. The loss of self-worth due to trauma is a real concern. This trust issue could make you afraid of anything and everything—new people, new places, new experiences, and so on. You may have won the battle with that traumatic moment, but anxiety is winning the war. Through applying my strategies later on in the book, you will eventually learn to regain this trust and love yourself once again.

Children

Though I assume that you yourself are no longer a child, this chapter wouldn't be complete if I didn't address the next generation and anxiety. We are seeing unprecedented rates of anxiety in children. And imagine being told as a kid that the only way you will ever feel better is to take medication. For the rest of your life, you feel that either someone or some substance is more equipped at helping you through tough situations than yourself.

Sometimes, medication is the only choice a parent has to help their child, and I don't blame them at all. I completely understand how helpful medication can be when struggling with real, debilitating symptoms. However, instead of looking at it as the end solution, we need to start considering it as a good stepping stone. These are life-altering choices we are making for our children because there just isn't a better option.

Why are so many children these days dealing with anxiety? I talked earlier about how trauma gives rise to anxiety. Most children have not yet experienced many traumas. Of course, there are unfortunately many children currently experiencing trauma, but there are also many more who have an incredibly loving upbringing and yet are more anxious than most adults. So this piece of the puzzle, when understanding the rise in anxiety, doesn't quite fit. What's going on?

Every age of development brings about different triggers to anxiety. For example, an infant or toddler may feel anxious and upset simply because they are overtired or hungry. They do not have the words to ask for food, or to say they need to rest, so they have an outburst attempting to relay the message that something is wrong and they don't know what. Anxiety is the response to a spidey sense alert trying to inform us that "hey, something isn't right—please do something about it."

There is a lot going on in a child. Children of any age are going through two massive changes: biological growth and neurological programming. They are learning how to walk, talk, eat, speak a language, read, and write. At the same time, children are also learning the unspoken nuances of this world, not to mention that the younger the child is, the more sensitive to energies they are. They pick up on and feel the energy between their parents and their peers. All children are empaths, though as they get older, those intuitions and feelings get suppressed. Kids are not yet aware of social norms, identities, and boundaries. Many of our human interactions are not consciously defined, and they are definitely not taught.

Outside influences can also have a larger effect on a kid. As we get older, our sense of self becomes more defined. For instance, as an adult, if you meet someone whose favorite color is red and yours is blue, it doesn't affect you; you've already committed yourself to your own tastes and you recognize that other people have their own ideas and preferences. However, as a child, there are none of these separations. Everything is coming at you at once with no idea how to process or interpret all of the information.

That said, children have always been this way, and there's always been a lot going on for them, so what is it that's changed to cause such huge rates of anxiety? Back in the day, children had the space and time to sit in boredom and process all the information they took on from school, from home, and from their own spidey senses. These days, whenever a child is bored or begins to whine, a parent is eager to stick a device in their face to quiet them down and keep them occupied. We are teaching our children at a very young age to suppress feelings through distraction.

There is already a lot going on for children both biologically and energetically. Then you add in an infinite amount of toys, along with TV shows and iPads. (The same way algorithms have enticed fully developed adult brains, the Netflixes and YouTube Kids of the world have done the same for children.) Because they are kept distracted, children are not getting a chance to process the influx of data. They are the oversaturated sponge to the max. I'll dive deeper into overstimulation in a different chapter because it's a significant source of anxiety for adults as well. For now, if you're a parent reading this, I urge you to minimize stimulation as much as possible in your child's life. While balance and moderation are important, I can assure you that even what we consider "minimal" within the context of today's world is already more than enough for their needs. Simplifying their environment and limiting screen time can make a profound difference for your empathic, oversaturated, anxious child.

Final Notes

With the increasing solar flares hitting our planet, more and more people are feeling restless and unsettled, like something is off, but they can't quite put their finger on it. Anxiety rates are skyrocketing every year, and yet no one seems to be understanding why. We're handed coping tools, medication, and mindfulness techniques, but we're rarely given a real explanation for what's actually happening beneath the surface.

Empaths, children, and trauma survivors are just three of the many groups most deeply affected, but anxiety doesn't stop there. It touches almost everyone in some way.

That's why, before we dive into solutions, I needed to lay out this foundation. You deserve to know why you feel this way and who is most affected by anxiety, because understanding these elements will make all the difference in how you heal.

Anxiety is rooted in everything, from childhood trauma to neurological processing and energetic sensitivity. There are layers upon layers of reasons why it manifests, making it impossible to point to a single, simple cause.

No, this book is not about quick fixes; **it's about reclaiming your power.** Healing anxiety requires knowledge and then action. It asks you to live differently, to observe yourself in ways you never have before, and to make choices that might feel uncomfortable at first. But I promise you this: If you're willing to do the work, this approach will change your life as it has mine. You've come to the right place—your intuition led you to this moment, to this book, to this next step in your journey. It's time to release it all; it's time to stop suppressing and start processing. So let's get to it. The real work begins now.

Key Chapter Takeaways

- Anxiety impacts highly sensitive people, trauma survivors, and children the most.
- Anxiety is an energy signal, and those who feel energy more will be more impacted by the signals. When

the signals go unnoticed, they can build, creating the oversaturated sponge.

- You need an energetic, subconscious, and vibrational approach to truly master anxiety long-term.

Key Action Steps

- Take the Oversaturated Sponge Quiz: Are you absorbing energy that isn't yours?
- Reflect on yourself as an empath. Do you feel more sensitive than others? How does that impact your day-to-day?
- List three ways you distract yourself from anxiety.

Client Case Study
John the Anxious Empath Who Didn't Know He Was One

John had been anxious for as long as he could remember, but not in the way that people could see: no panic attacks, no dramatic breakdowns. His anxiety was a constant background hum of unease that followed him everywhere. He tried therapy, medication, and mindfulness retreats but nothing seemed to help. If anything, he felt worse.

When we started working together, I asked him, "How long have you been feeling this way?"

John exhaled sharply as he responded, "Honestly? I don't know life without it. It's just always been there." The confusing part for him was that everything in his childhood had been good. From the outside, some would even say he had the perfect upbringing. But I started digging a little deeper.

"Did you feel safe to express how you were really feeling?" I asked.

He paused for a moment. "I mean, I didn't have big feelings, or at least . . . I don't think I did."

"Did anyone ever ask?" I said gently.

This clearly struck something in him because there was a longer pause this time before he responded, "No. Everyone just expected me to be okay, and I was. I had to be."

It was this conversation that began unraveling the threads affecting him from childhood. We began putting the pieces together. It wasn't what *happened* to John that affected him; it was the underlying energies from childhood that did.

When he was growing up, his parents weren't openly fighting, but there was this tension in the air, a constant feeling of unease that would never seem to go away. No yelling, no big traumatic moments, just this heavy, silent weight. I explained to him, "This tension you felt was energy, and as a sensitive, empathic kid, you felt everything. You picked up on all of it, even if no one spoke a word, and you haven't put it down since."

Something strong had clearly clicked in him. He looked down at his hands as he said, "So it's not just in my head?"

"No, John, it's not. You were never the problem; you were just the sponge." I had to explain to him that when you're a natural feeler, and no one teaches you how to process all that energy, you learn to doubt yourself instead.

John had spent his whole life feeling things no one else acknowledged, which made him think that *he* was the problem. Once he realized his anxiety wasn't his fault, and that it was simply an energetic overload, everything shifted. We used my ReNU technique to heal the subconscious wounds of not being seen or understood, then applied Vibrational Navigation so he could finally separate his emotions from the ones he absorbed from others. (I'll cover both ReNU and Vibrational Navigation in chapter five.)

The result was incredible. For the first time in years, John felt in control. His anxiety wasn't gone, but it had a purpose now—it was a signal, not a curse. His sleep improved, his brain fog cleared, and he stopped feeling at war with himself. If you, like John, have ever felt anxious for no reason, constantly questioning why you're overwhelmed when everything in your life seems fine, you need to know this: You're not crazy; you're just feeling more energy than most people. With the techniques we'll cover in later chapters, you, too, can feel the shift.

Chapter 3

Unfinished Business: Anxiety and the Past

Hey Anxiety Ally,

Do you wake up and already feel overwhelmed? Do simple tasks, like laundry or running errands, feel like monumental challenges? Even when you're doing something you love, do you find yourself unable to shake a sense of restlessness or unease?

If this resonates with you, here's something to think about: The anxiety you're experiencing has nothing to do with the present moment. Yes, the world feels chaotic, but that's not the true source of these feelings. For many of us, anxiety stems from something deeper. Maybe it's the survival mode we've been living in for years, conditioned to just get by as a way to stay safe. Maybe it's the defense mechanisms that served us in the past but now feel like they're stuck in overdrive. Your anxiety is being driven by things in the past.

While this might be the way it had to be, it's not the way it has to stay. This isn't just about managing anxiety. It's about uncovering the reasons behind it, reconnecting with your inner calm, and creating a life where you can thrive, not just survive. You don't have to carry this weight alone. **It's time to give your overworked defense systems the rest they deserve and reclaim the joy and peace that's always been yours.**

Anxiety in Time

In order to heal from anxiety long term, we must first observe and then neutralize the cause of the anxiety itself. Once again, previous anxiety solutions have failed all of us because they focus on symptoms and only ever provide limited relief. As I went deeper into exploring the root cause of my clients' anxiety, and my own, I began seeing the theme of *time* pop up. Yes, time. I know it sounds weird, but stay with me. It seemed like anxiety showed up differently depending on whether I was observing it through the past, the present, or the future. The root cause of the spidey sense alert would change. So, instead of attempting to understand every person's individual situation, and every *exact* cause, I began finding that if we could determine what *direction* the anxiety was coming from, it was much easier to find sustainable solutions that actually worked.

Think about a layer of anxiety existing in each of these time frames. In order to sustainably heal from anxiety, we need to peel back each layer. It would be so nice to say that everyone has just one area of their lives to focus on in order to end the cycle of anxiety, but that's just not the case. If you're anything like me, you will have to explore the past, present, and future in order to truly get a handle on your mind. Along the way, you will learn so much about who you are and what you are capable of. **Besides, anxiety is your intuition's way of reminding you just how powerful you are.**

The past is the most dominant source of anyone's anxiety, and for good reason. The emotional traumas of humanity have been ignored for many years. As a collective, we have been thrown into generations of suffering and survival. That means that no one had the time or energy to care if they hurt your feelings growing up; there were more difficult situations at hand. Remember, World War I ended just over one hundred years ago. It wasn't until the end of the Baby Boomer years, and the beginnings of Generation X's and Millennials' time, where the conversation and fear around war had ceased.

The reason I bring this up is because the majority of us have never been taught how to actually navigate our emotions. These days are different, and parenting approaches are starting to catch up. (I'm teaching my son meditation and breathing techniques at just a year and a half old.) Although I would hope all Millennial and Gen Z parents teach their kids this level of emotional intelligence and mindfulness, I know that most aren't. Their parents never taught them, and their grandparents never taught their parents. What I'm really getting at here is that most of us suffer from trauma and lack of emotional regulation because no one gave us the tools to properly process unresolved emotions. I believe that most individuals with chronic anxiety are suffering from past traumas that are currently affecting them. When anxiety pops up from the present or the future, its symptoms are different than signs of anxiety from the past.

Past anxiety has everything to do with the buildup of energies going unresolved, which makes you an oversaturated sponge. If you really think about it, many of the actions we take in our lives could be divided into two categories: taking action on something new, or maintaining something old. Our life is filled with rudimentary maintenance tasks. Dirty laundry, for example, builds up to the point where you finally have to wash it—that's maintaining something old. Just buying new clothes, on the other hand, would be taking action on something new. In fact, most of our days and weeks are directed toward maintenance: answering emails in your inbox, taking a shower, refilling your water bottle, washing the dishes, adding gas to your car, and so on.

But while it's easy to wash the dishes when we see that they are dirty in the sink, it's not as easy to see a pile of unresolved emotions sitting inside ourselves, especially when we are skilled at disassociating and are never given the tools to know how to clear them. Energetic maintenance is just as, if not more, important than physical maintenance, and yet no one has taught us how.

Imagine putting on a layer of clothing, and then another one, and another one. You eventually keep adding layers until you can't move, see, or even breathe. This is what unresolved emotional layers do to us on the inside. We get to a point where we are so overwhelmed, we can't handle one more addition. It is only when a panic attack hits that we recognize that something needs to change and seek professional help. Once we have finally had enough, the professional we seek out gives us a pill that makes us numb to feeling any of the layers. Until, of course, the pill wears off and the overwhelm creeps back in. We need to learn to peel back that layer of past anxiety so that we can live free of the burden of unresolved feelings. See if either of the following symptoms of past anxiety feels true to your experience.

Chronic Dis-ease and Recurrent Anxiety

People who wake up and continuously feel a sense of dis-ease or restlessness are most likely dealing with unresolved energies and emotions from the past. As an oversaturated sponge, you have taken on, and taken on, and taken on, and are now existing in a constant breaking point all throughout your day and week. Your spidey sense alarm bells are ringing nonstop. Every once in a while something small happens, and it's that critical "one thing too much"; you have a breakdown, and feel better for a couple of days or even weeks, until the restlessness and buildup continues.

Dis-ease: The imbalance that occurs when we fall out of alignment, allowing lower vibrations like fear, stress, or resistance to manifest physically, emotionally, or spiritually.

A lot of the time, when we feel this way, we make big life decisions thinking that they will resolve the chronic tension.

This is where some major, long-term loops get started. Imagine this: You wake up one morning with a heavy feeling in your chest. It's not entirely unfamiliar, but today, it's louder than it usually is. You feel uneasy, restless, and a little trapped. You sit with that discomfort for a while and your mind starts to run, trying to figure out what's wrong. It doesn't take long for it to land on your job. After all, you've been dealing with some tough situations at work lately—maybe your boss hasn't been as supportive as you'd like or you've been feeling undervalued, or the workload has been overwhelming. It clicks in your mind: *This must be why I feel this way—it's the job that's the problem.* The moment you link your anxiety to your job, it feels like a solution is within reach. You just need to change jobs, and you'll feel better. Suddenly, the anxious energy propels you into action. You polish up your résumé, spend hours scrolling through job listings, and send out applications. The anxiety starts to shift into something more productive, even exciting. Every job interview feels like a step closer to freedom, and when you finally get an offer and accept it, relief washes over you. You tell yourself, *This is it; this new job is going to change everything. I'm finally going to feel better.*

And for a little while, it works. The excitement of starting fresh, learning new things, and meeting new people is invigorating. That sense of relief lasts for a few months, and you convince yourself that you made the right call. But then, without warning, the old, familiar anxiety starts creeping back in. It's subtle at first, just a nagging feeling of unease. You ignore it, distract yourself, and tell yourself it's nothing, but it doesn't go away; it just grows louder and more persistent, and soon, you're right back where you started—restless, anxious, and searching for an explanation. This time, maybe you blame something else. Maybe it's your relationship, your city, or even your apartment that feels wrong. Once again, you latch on to a solution, make another big change. And the anxiety will go away—until it doesn't—and the cycle continues.

I know about this cycle because I have been in it myself, and witnessed it in others often. It's something that happens a lot within romantic relationships; couples might decide to have a baby, move houses, get married, or adopt a pet in hopes that those big life changes will solve their problems. It's a doubling-down effect. Of course, piling on more responsibilities will only ever create more anxiety. **Trying to address our anxiety—whether we think we're finding a solution or simply a distraction from the feeling—we subconsciously create *more* problems we'll have to solve.** And people live their entire lives like this, never actually being able to solve the anxiety for good.

If we don't dig deep and go into our past, we won't be able to fully show up in the present. The majority of chronic anxiety comes down to a buildup of unresolved energies that are triggering our spidey sense alarm constantly. We use food, and shopping, and social media, and sometimes drugs or alcohol to cover up these alarms because we don't have the tools to turn them off.

Does this resonate with you? Have you found yourself stuck in these "doubling-down" loops before? Do you still have bouts of low-level anxiety you can't seem to shake? Well, once you understand where the emotional buildup is coming from, and then take the time to heal it, you will be able to free yourself for good.

Fear Preventing Movement

The other symptom of past anxiety I want to explore is the fear of movement. **Essentially, when we are living in a state with layers and layers of energy built up, it prevents us from being able to show up in the present moment and make decisions that will allow us to move forward.** Our drive to try new things is stifled by an internal dialogue riddled with fear and insecurity. Unresolved childhood bullying could lead you to a life of seeking validation and perfection. Unresolved financial traumas could lead you to a life of either overspending or hoarding your money. Unresolved abuse could lead you to a life of either over-trusting others and giving your power away, or never trusting anyone and lying to create safety. When you pile up all the unresolved emotions and situations from your entire life, there are a lot of dynamics at play. This is why, as we get older, anxieties tend to increase because there are more unresolved emotions we need to heal.

Over time, we end up losing trust in ourselves to make the right decision and we lose trust in the world for supporting us when we need it the most. This lack of trust inherently prevents us from exploring new things. **Our subconscious mind gives us reasons why we need to fear new experiences.** All of the alarm bells are going off, so in order to feel safe or protected, it's easiest to just stay in the same place. It's safer to eat the same food, travel to the same destinations, and surround yourself with the same people. Even if it's not the best choice, we have the knowledge and tools to navigate the expected outcomes. When we are in survival mode, we do not have the extra energy or awareness to navigate new scenarios, and if we are thrown into one unexpectedly, then all hell breaks loose on the inside.

Sometimes, if our subconscious mind is unable to find the cause of the alarm, it will choose something random and identify it as the problem. The reason why our minds do this automatically is because they are *designed* to solve problems, and if they don't understand the root cause of the problem, they cannot solve it. An example of this mechanism can be seen in people with specific phobias, like a fear of heights or spiders. On a subconscious level, their mind directs their anxiety into a single, tangible target, creating an intense fear and aversion to that thing. While this may seem counterproductive, it actually provides some relief from the constant, overwhelming tension of general anxiety. By hyper-focusing on one specific fear, they are able to compartmentalize their anxiety, allowing them to function in other areas of life. For instance, someone with a fear of spiders can still grocery shop or navigate most of their day without that fear interfering. This highlights how the mind often seeks ways to manage anxiety, either by creating a general state of hyperawareness or by fixating on one specific cause. Both approaches serve as coping mechanisms to handle the persistent buildup of lingering emotional energy. However, whether the focus is broad or specific, the underlying anxiety is still rooted in old, unresolved energy that needs to be untangled and addressed at its source.

Healing the Past

So how do you go about unzipping all of those layers, squeezing the water out of that sponge, and finally releasing the unseen tension tearing through your body and mind? Remember, healing is a journey, and one that never truly ends. Just because you've washed the dishes, that doesn't mean you never need to wash them again. **As we experience life, energies and emotions come up, and constant maintenance is required to feel balance and alignment.**

The hardest part is always starting at the beginning, which is healing the past. As we move through the layers on to the present and future, things get easier. If you don't do the work on your past, your chronic anxiety will not go away—it's as simple as that.

Although I wish simply reading this chapter would magically heal you, it's definitely not that simple. It takes a long time to heal from old wounds. However, if you are just starting this journey, there is some good news: What used to take many years is now being expedited. Due to the increasing energy on planet Earth, our healing is happening rapidly. Besides, the only reason why energies and emotions stuck with you in the first place is that you never gave yourself enough time to *process them.* **Once you are in a place willing to show up and feel it all, healing can really start to take place.** So, if you're hesitating, know that now is the perfect time to start.

First, it's important to be aware of how affected you are by the past. Many of you have done a lot of work on yourselves, so it can be tricky just hopping in without knowing where you are. Let's go through a little evaluation quiz in order to determine where you sit on your healing journey so that you can better understand where to go from here.

Quiz: How Healed Are You from Past Traumas?

Instructions: Answer each question with a simple "Yes" or "No." For every "Yes," give yourself 1 point. At the end, tally your score to see where you stand on your healing journey.

1. Do you often feel anxious in situations where there's no immediate threat?
2. Do you often find yourself replaying past events or conversations in your mind?
3. Do certain memories still trigger intense emotional reactions?
4. Do you struggle with trusting others due to past experiences?
5. Do you notice patterns of self-sabotage in your relationships or goals?
6. Do you feel unworthy or undeserving of happiness or success?
7. Do you avoid situations or people that remind you of past pain?
8. Do you often feel overwhelmed by emotions you can't fully explain?
9. Do you have difficulty staying present in the

moment, frequently worrying about the future or dwelling on the past?

10. Do you feel like you haven't fully processed certain events from your past?

Your Score & Results

0–3 Points: Healed and Empowered

Congratulations! You've done significant work to heal from your past traumas. While no one is ever fully "finished" healing, you are in a strong place where past events have little control over your present. Keep nurturing your growth and self-awareness.

4–7 Points: Healing in Progress

You've made progress, but there are still areas where past traumas may be influencing your current feelings, including anxiety. Focus on understanding the root causes of these emotions and seek some additional tools and suggestions in this chapter.

8–10 Points: Healing Needed

Your score suggests that unresolved past traumas may be significantly impacting your emotional well-being. This could be contributing to your current anxiety and limiting your ability to fully experience life. It's time to prioritize deep healing work through supportive methods mentioned in the coming pages.

You may either be pleasantly surprised by your score, or shocked at how unhealed you may be. No matter where you sit, you're currently in a really good place because you are reading this. By picking up this book you made a choice, a choice to no longer feel imprisoned by your own mind. If you scored 8–10, you need to take some serious time digging into past traumas and **heal them through feeling them**. It doesn't mean that you can't read the rest of the book, but it does mean that after you finish this book, you need to start taking action on purging what no longer serves you. Ideally, you will know you're healed completely when you can connect to painful past experiences with no negative emotional reaction. Eventually, by addressing the past, present, and future aspects of anxiety, you may be able to look into your previous traumas and actually feel a sense of gratitude toward them.

For over a decade, I have worked with clients to help them heal their traumas and reclaim control over their lives. There are a variety of different healing methods available to you—acupuncture, Reiki, past life regression, therapy, meditation, Rife machines . . . I could go on and on. There are three techniques I'm going to focus on here because they were the ones that had the biggest impact on me and my clients, and you can do them yourself. Keep in mind, this book isn't about healing your past traumas; it's about healing anxiety. Healing in and of itself is a journey, one that will deeply help your chronic anxiety, but you have to be willing to take the lead if you want the change.

Sitting with It

It seems like we just never have enough time. Everything and everyone demands your attention. When you're at work and a wave of sadness suddenly hits you, what do you do? Most of us just push it down. There never seems to be a good time in the day to stop and fully feel. When you finally do get a quiet moment, all you want to do is veg out on the couch and binge-watch some terrible reality TV. We barely have time to shower every day, let alone find the time to just sit and do nothing but feel.

I get the reality of life, but it's this very reality that's fueling our anxiety. Instead of sweeping everything under the rug, what if we gave ourselves permission to sit and feel? We live in a constant loop of reacting to life instead of witnessing it. When we don't make space for our emotions in the present, they don't just disappear—they pile up. That buildup then creates emotional clutter we're forced to sort through later.

Sitting with your emotions isn't easy. It requires courage and vulnerability. But when you feel something and you actually allow yourself to sit with it, without judgment, without needing to change it, something powerful happens: The emotion starts to shift, and over time, the intensity softens. Eventually, you'll notice that something that used to trigger you doesn't anymore. That's your cue that you're ready to go deeper and look at the roots, at what's still hiding beneath the surface.

It doesn't take much to clear out the old energies, but it does take presence. Find a safe, quiet space like your bedroom, your car, or a bench in nature, close your eyes, and breathe. Gently clear the noise of the present moment. Then, let yourself travel back to the moments that still feel painful. Observe the memory and allow the emotions to move through you. Take slow, rhythmic breaths as you do this. Sometimes, your nervous system will sound the alarm, telling you that you're unsafe. That's okay; just remind yourself you *are* safe now. Stay with the memory and allow yourself to feel all of it. Cry if the tears come. Laugh or yell if you need to. The point is to create space for what was never fully processed. As you revisit the same memory with the awareness of safety, the emotional charge starts to dissolve. Do this as many times as you need. Afterward, you might want to call a friend, write in a journal, or talk to a therapist. Sometimes we need support to help us process what's been stored.

Sitting with your emotions doesn't mean fixing, analyzing, or judging them. It just means showing up. It means being curious about the parts of yourself that have lived in the shadows. And here's the real shift: Anxiety isn't the enemy; it's a signal. It's your system asking for your awareness. By sitting with your unresolved emotions, you're essentially saying, "I hear you, and I'm ready to turn off the alarm before it needs to sound."

Talking to Yourself

Talking to yourself might sound silly or even a little crazy. Society has taught us that people who talk to themselves are unstable or need help, but in reality, self-talk is one of the most powerful tools for self-healing. Our minds are incredibly busy, constantly reacting to the world, processing emotions, and planning actions. If we don't stop and pay attention to what's happening internally, it's like letting a storm rage on. Believe it or not, before we say something out loud, our minds are already planning the words. Our thoughts move so quickly that we don't usually catch the internal dialogue happening underneath the surface. **But when we take the time to listen, we can uncover the emotions driving our reactions.**

For example, before I ask my partner to cut up our toddler Bodhi's food, I feel a sense of panic or fear about him choking. That fear leads me to act, prompting me to speak up and ask her to cut the food. On the surface, it might look like I'm being overly controlling, but if I dig deeper, I realize that the fear is tied to trust issues stemming from past traumas—traumas that aren't even connected to food or choking, which is where things can get confusing. These anxieties create external loops where I feel the need to control a situation in order to avoid my worst fears coming true. We all have these subtle mechanisms playing out in the background of our lives, usually without realizing it. The key to breaking these loops is stopping the pattern in its tracks through talking to yourself.

In my case, I might pause and turn inward, asking myself, *Hey, Liz, how are you feeling right now? Why are you scared?* When I did this recently, I discovered that, earlier in the day, my partner had forgotten to put on Bodhi's helmet while he was riding his bicycle, and he fell. It wasn't a bad fall, but it triggered a feeling of insecurity in me. By addressing this part of myself directly, while bringing awareness to the cause of my dis-ease, I could acknowledge the fear and allow it to surface instead of letting it unconsciously drive my actions.

Sometimes, these check-ins don't even require spoken words. I might ask myself how I'm feeling and suddenly feel a wave of sadness or tears welling up. Instead of trying to rationalize it or figure out the "why," I just let myself cry and sit with the emotion. It's so important to give yourself space to feel. In a fast-paced world, scheduling an hour a week for emotions isn't enough. You need to check in with yourself throughout the day.

Here's another example: One night I was relaxing, watching Netflix, when I suddenly felt like I couldn't catch my breath. My chest tightened, and I started sweating—classic signs of an impending panic attack. I tried deep breathing and safety affirmations, but they weren't working. So, instead, I turned inward and asked myself, *Hey, Liz, what's going on? Are you okay?* The voice that came back was quiet and shaky and said, *There's just so much going on.* It wasn't one specific thing; it was everything: the chaos in the world, bills that needed paying, chores that were piling up. So I responded gently, *It is a lot, and that's okay. Right now, there's nothing you need to do. You have all the tools needed to handle the rest.* That simple conversation created the validation that it *was* a lot and that it was *okay.* My body relaxed, my breath slowed, and the cold sweats stopped.

When we talk to ourselves this way, we become our own caretakers. **We show up for ourselves in ways that no one else ever has before, fostering trust and communication with the parts of us that feel scared or unheard.** This not only helps us heal, it also builds a self-awareness that allows us to understand our reactions on a deeper level. If you want to go even further, try checking in with yourself before you fall asleep at night. Ask yourself how your day went and if there was any big emotion or reaction you need to process. This daily check-in will help you sleep more deeply since your mind won't be trying to process unresolved energies on its own. It will also allow you to wake up ready to start a new day without the baggage of the previous day lingering.

Cord-Cutting Letter

The third technique is to write a cord-cutting letter. Before we dive into what that is, let me briefly describe what an energetic cord is first. An energy cord is an invisible emotional or energetic link formed between you and objects, people, or experiences you interact with. Every interaction we have creates energetic connections or cords. These cords affect everything from your emotions to your thoughts and reactions. Energy cannot usually be seen by the naked eye, but it can be felt, as long as we are listening. Most cords are weak and dissipate naturally, but intense emotional attachments form stronger ones. These strong cords *can* eventually release over time once there is a separation between you and whatever you connected with, but they can also linger. When we move through life and go through countless daily interactions, the energy cords build up. The more cords you have, the more anxiety you are bound to feel. Once again, it's like adding layer after layer of clothing only to get to a point where you feel utterly stifled and claustrophobic. Releasing or cutting these cords is an extremely important tool for anxiety management.

Energetic Cord: An invisible emotional or energetic link formed between you and objects, people, or experiences you interact with, influencing your thoughts and feelings.

Cord Cutting: The intentional practice of severing unhealthy or unwanted attachments to people, entities, past experiences, or timelines. It frees your energy body from draining connections, restores sovereignty, and allows for higher vibrational alignment with your soul's path.

Energy Body: The subtle, nonphysical layer of yourself that senses and processes energetic information from the environment before your physical brain becomes aware.

Cord cutting can be done through the following methods:

- Simple cords can be cleared with water. Showering, bathing, or washing your hands and allowing the water to absorb the energy from the cord is excellent for cleansing minor attachments.
- Having a crystal nearby (such as selenite or amethyst) or burning white sage can help to clear energetic connections.

- You can simply visualize a cord between you and whatever is pulling your energy and then visualize yourself cutting that cord with a pair of scissors.
- Stronger attachments can be cleared by writing a cord-cutting letter.

I want to lay out the cord-cutting letter method to help you heal and move forward. The reason for writing a letter is to identify and address the past trauma, but then to also *feel* how that affects you emotionally in the present. It targets both the structured logical side, as well as the empathic and emotional side of us. Essentially, it gives you all the components needed for release and healing old, stuck energies. Even if you have done this before, it may be time to do it again.

This letter needs to be written out by hand rather than typed—it's more impactful that way. The letter can be short or long; it really doesn't matter, as long as you truly take the time to feel each word. You can write individual letters addressing individual situations or people. Or you can address multiple traumas at once, in one big letter. Keep in mind that you will not be sending this letter to anyone—you will be destroying it at the end, in order to release it for good.

Once you start your letter, you can take your time on it, stopping and coming back when needed. If you cry, laugh, or get angry when writing it, that's a good thing. Allow any and all emotions to flow. The more you feel when writing it, the more you are releasing and healing the past.

I've put together a structure for the letter on the next page. Please take your time writing out and answering each question, and add in anything else you may feel the need to write. Once again, this letter is holding space for big emotions, so make sure you show up for yourself and feel it all while writing.

Cord-Cutting Letter Structure

- What was the situation that created the trauma (who did it involve, how old were you, and so on)?
- How did that make you feel emotionally?
- If you could say anything to that person or people without repercussion, what would it be?
- If you could say anything to your past self from back in that time, what would it be?
- What did you learn from those experiences?
- Write a line or two of forgiveness toward yourself.
- Write a line or two of forgiveness toward others in the letter who hurt you.
- After all is said and done, what are you the most grateful for in the aftermath of those situations?
- A final sentence to close: "I clear any and all trauma, emotions, and contracts with the people and situations above, for the highest good of all involved."

Once you have addressed all of those questions in your letter, you are ready to let it go for good. Take the letter, read it over one final time, feel everything it brings up, and find a safe place to burn it. There is something uniquely powerful about burning that helps clear emotions.

After writing and burning the letter, you'll likely start to feel shifts almost immediately. Sometimes this process can stir things up, making it seem like life is getting harder. People may suddenly exit your life, or you might experience a sudden change, like losing a job you've had for years. It's important to recognize that these changes are a natural part of the clearing process. What's leaving you is tied to the old energy you just released and it no longer aligns with who you are becoming. By writing this letter and diving deep into your past to release what no longer serves you, you are making a conscious choice to change. And with that decision, old aspects of your life will naturally fall away, creating space for new opportunities to emerge. Embrace the transformation, knowing that what's ahead is in greater alignment with your highest good.

Final Notes

I think we all know that the only constant in life is change itself. When we haven't taken the time to look into the past and feel it all, it will eventually catch up to us. Old energies build and build until we become the oversaturated sponge and simply don't have the capacity to hold anything new. When we end up carrying all of the weight from old traumas and emotions, our spidey sense alert is constantly ringing. When we are in this state, we become hypervigilant to the point where all of our systems are stretched to their limit. There isn't just one cause of our anxiety—it's all of the past, all at once. The more we ignore these signals with distractions, the worse it ends up getting, until we hit a breaking point. **You have to break down before you break through.** Well, if you haven't already broken through, then this is your time. If you scored 8–10 points in the healing quiz, then I recommend you take a break before the next chapter and write out your cord-cutting letter. It's time for you to access freedom in your mind and body, and in order to do that, you must release what you've been carrying—it no longer serves you, and it's preventing you from moving forward in all areas. I just want to say, I'm proud of you, and you should be proud of yourself too!

Key Chapter Takeaways

- Unprocessed emotions accumulate like layers, making anxiety feel constant.
- The process of healing yourself can look as simple as creating the space and time to sit and talk to yourself about any thoughts or feelings that may be going unnoticed.
- Most chronic anxiety stems from unresolved past experiences rather than present issues.

Key Action Steps

- Take the "How Healed Are You from Past Traumas?" quiz.
- Sit with an old memory that triggers anxiety, and instead of suppressing it, allow yourself to feel it with the reminder of safety.
- Write out a cord-cutting letter recognizing the past traumas and releasing them with forgiveness and gratitude.
- Take the time to talk to yourself and check in; it will create a sense of trust and build strong foundations for the future.

Client Case Study
Mike: The High-Functioning Anxiety Trap

Mike was incredibly successful. He had a solid career, he was a great dad, and he was loved by everyone around him. But inside, he was breaking. Anxiety had been creeping up on him for years, and he had no idea why. He convinced himself that it was just work stress, but deep down, he knew that wasn't the full story. When we first spoke, he laughed off the idea of anxiety. "I've never had a panic attack or anything," he told me. "I just get irritated . . . snappy, even, when there's no reason to be."

I nodded. "And what about sleep?"

"Terrible," he said with a sigh. "I wake up at 3 AM like clockwork and can't get my mind to settle long enough to go back to sleep, then I'm just tired all day." He paused, rubbed his temples, and went on, "I don't even know why—my life is good. I *should* feel fine."

That's when I turned the tables on him. "Mike, maybe the problem isn't your life. Maybe it's about what you've never let yourself *feel*?"

Here's what was actually happening: **Mike had never been taught how to feel.** Growing up, emotions equaled weakness. When I asked him if he was taught how to regulate emotions in childhood, he chuckled and responded with, "We didn't talk about feelings.

When I was growing up, my dad would say, 'If you're not bleeding, you're fine.' In his family, men didn't talk about their feelings—they sucked it up and moved on." So that's exactly what he did.

"Emotions don't just vanish because we ignore them, Mike. They pile up like unprocessed files in the background slowing down your systems and clogging your clarity. It's completely normal for you to feel a constant sense of irritability with such a weight on your shoulders, a weight you weren't even aware of." He had never considered this. I told him, "If you don't deal with them, they get stored in your body, and eventually they explode and take the form of chronic anxiety, irritability, exhaustion, and even physical symptoms like headaches and insomnia."

Mike's anxiety wasn't about his job or his responsibilities; it was about decades of suppressed emotions demanding to be felt. So I did what no one had ever taught him how to do: feel them completely. Through guided reflection, self-talk, and cord-cutting, we released everything he had buried for years. And yeah, it was uncomfortable at first, but then it was freeing. For the first time, his anxiety started to fade, not because he "got rid of it," but because he sat with it. Mike stopped just getting through life and actually started living it. Now he's a different man: He's present with his kids, engaged with his relationships, and finally feels like himself again.

So if you've ever felt like you're doing everything "right" but still feel restless, on edge, or exhausted, ask yourself, "What have I been avoiding feeling?" Trust me, it's not your job, or your schedule. It's the emotional weight you've been carrying from the past, and you don't have to carry it anymore.

Chapter 4

Drowning in Vibes: Navigating Present Anxiety

Hey Anxiety Ally,

Do you ever feel like throwing in the towel? Like no matter how hard you try, there's always this underlying sense of overwhelm lurking in the background? The house never stays clean, the bills seem endless, and let's not even get started on the constant doomscroll of global catastrophes. Every headline feels like another brick added to the weight you're carrying.

On top of all this chaos, we're becoming more energetically sensitive. As discussed back in chapter two, phenomena like solar flares affect the electromagnetic frequency around us, and these energetic shifts seem to amplify everything. Suddenly, paying bills isn't just paying bills anymore. It's feeling the weight of inflation, financial uncertainty, and the future of the economy all rolled into one.

We are no longer living in a simple, transactional world. The layers of the physical, emotional, and energetic world just keep piling up. It's no wonder we're all feeling maxed out. But hey, you're not alone in this, and there are ways to cut through the noise, take control, and start feeling better.

In this chapter, we're going to tackle the overstimulation of modern life head-on. From clearing out the external inputs that weigh us down, to embracing tools like cold showers and purposeful discomfort, this is where we start reclaiming our peace. No matter how loud the world gets, we've got this, and we've got each other, so let's figure it out together.

Anxiety Is Contagious

The title of this book says it all: Your anxiety is giving me anxiety. Unlike anxiety from the past, which is caused by unresolved emotions and trauma, anxiety from the present is coming from outside of us. In the present, there are a myriad of triggers that will set off our spidey sense alerts—the *root cause* of our anxiety. One of the biggest triggers of the alarm is coming from our external world.

When we observe this world as a physical system with interactions that involve our five senses, it's easy to understand cause and effect. You smell a freshly baked croissant in the coffee shop, and you immediately feel hungry. Cause and effect. When we dive deep into the intrinsic energetic world and interactions that trigger our spidey sense, on the other hand, it can be difficult to figure out why we feel a certain way when we can't observe the direct cause of that feeling.

Let's go back to the example from chapter two, of going to the grocery store and feeling the energy from the cashier: In your logical mind, you simply went to the store to pick up a few things, bought them, and came home. There was nothing notable or significant about your time spent doing this chore. Meanwhile, you interacted with someone who was feeling a strong emotion and you ended up taking that emotion home with you. That emotion is not yours, and yet now you have it. In fact, I bet the cashier felt a little better after you left.

You see, it's not just anxiety that's contagious; all energy and emotion is. The busier our external world is, the more interactions we have, and therefore the more energy is exchanged. We don't just exchange energy with people but also with situations and external objects. For instance, getting stuck in traffic doesn't mean you're interacting with one specific person and picking up their energy, but the situation itself can still affect us emotionally. As another example, watching the news isn't a two-way conversation or in-person interaction, and yet, it still affects you. Maybe you watch news coverage of a war happening overseas and you see the displaced children on the screen. Your thoughts race and you just want someone to help them, or to at least hold them. If you're a parent, you might think of your own children and what they would go through in the same situation. All of these thoughts and emotions happen so quickly, your conscious mind doesn't have a chance to recognize them. After watching the news, the rest of the day feels off, you feel removed from your own life, or just sad and unmotivated to do anything. But you might not recognize that this feeling you have has come from watching the news earlier, so you can't pinpoint the cause of the emotion. Your mind starts to spiral, attempting to figure out what's wrong in order to prepare the best solution. Once again, the *cause* of anxiety is that spidey sense alert, and the *symptom* of it is your mind and body responding to the alert, attempting to solve an unseen issue.

Conscious Mind: The active, aware aspect of perception that processes thoughts, logic, and decision-making in real time.

The world around us prompts us to constantly engage, and within those interactions we are bombarded with energies we need to process. (This is why naturally anxious people often choose not to go out and do much, and if we do, we need at least a week or two to recover.) But because we have never been taught about the energetic connections around us, our minds only focus on perceived physical threats. **It's really the *confusion* about why the alarm is ringing that creates the majority of the anxiety symptoms.** When I began teaching my mind to solve problems by observing both the physical and nonphysical worlds, my anxiety began to decrease exponentially.

This chapter will explore the unseen connections around us and how to navigate them with ease. Remember, this book isn't going to stop the daily challenges of life, but instead, teach you how to navigate through them without any extra effort or anxiety. **Change is the constant, but how we respond to the change is everything.**

Before we move on: Let's assume you've already begun, or even completed (for now), the process of clearing out energy from the past. While it's possible to learn new techniques for managing present-moment anxiety while still carrying unresolved past issues, until the past is processed, you will continue looping back into old anxiety patterns. This is why addressing the past is essential for breaking the cycle and truly moving forward. If you haven't yet started the process I laid out in chapter three, I suggest you do it before getting started with this chapter's concepts.

Consumption Versus Creation

I recently realized that I was wasting a lot of time scrolling on Instagram, and I tried convincing myself that I needed to be on there because it was my main platform to reach people. But that justification didn't stick. When I found myself spending hours staring at my phone, I had to ask myself, "Am I creating or consuming at this moment?" and the answer, most of the time, was "consuming."

Then I needed to ask the follow-up question: "Is consuming this content benefiting my overall well-being?" And, not surprisingly, most of the time the answer was "no." I use this technique now as a check-in for myself. The question, "Am I creating or consuming?" is one that I believe we all need to ask ourselves.

As we consume more, we naturally stimulate ourselves

more. It could look like consuming content on YouTube, listening to podcasts, or binge-watching Netflix. But it could also be buying stuff we don't need from Amazon, eating that whole bag of chips, and so on. Think of consumption in your life as "input." When we input things into our minds, bodies, and souls, it has an effect on us, either negative or positive.

When we are inputting more than we are outputting, a sort of energetic traffic jam happens. Our minds and bodies can only handle so much input or consumption. Eventually there needs to be an output. Think of the oversaturated sponge example from chapter two. A dry sponge can only hold so much water before it gets to be too much and it all pours out. In an emotional sense, we can only handle so much emotional input before we need to cry, or talk it out, or otherwise output what we've been processing. In an ideal world, the consumption and creation ratio would match each other. It means you wouldn't have to hit the gym to work off the excess calories, or pay for therapy to release the excess emotion. **When we moderate the input and output, we feel healthy, balanced, and aligned.** It's like showing up to a clean kitchen to do some cooking. You feel free to move forward, rather than spending the time and energy cleaning up your previous mess.

Our current world is dominated by consumption, eating more, working more, spending more, and doing more. It never ends. I think so many of us become trapped in consumption, not only because society pushes it, but because it feels so good in the moment. Buying that thing, eating that thing, spending that money, scrolling for hours . . . all have been proven to release chemical compounds like dopamine and serotonin in the brain. The effect is like getting a hit of a new and potent drug. Eventually, we get used to the feeling and buying that one thing isn't enough to give us the same "hit," so we need to buy more. Or eat more, or consume more pointless videos on TikTok, and so on. **Consuming overstimulates our physical and mental bodies, leading to overwhelm—and, therefore, anxiety.**

When we do choose to create something instead of consume, it's not as rapidly rewarding. It takes time, patience, presence, and focus to take action. Making a meal is a great example of creating. Recording a video rather than watching one is a great example of output rather than input. Of course, when we make food, we get to enjoy both the creation and consumption. Similarly, creating a business takes a lot of time, hard work, and dedication, but eventually you'll be able to enjoy the financial benefits and consume what you've created.

These days, so many of us want that immediate dopamine hit rather than taking the time to create. **When we aren't actively creating our reality through focus and action, we feel unfulfilled and stuck, and, of course, anxious.**

So what's the solution? Balance. Take a hard look at your life and day-to-day. How much output versus input do you participate in? Then ask yourself, "Of the output, how much of it is for myself and how much is for others?" When you drive around and pick your kids up, cook them dinner, go to work, and answer your emails, that's all technically for others. When you take a bath, or write in your journal, or set intentions around what you want to manifest, that is all output directed toward *yourself*.

In a lot of ways, distracting ourselves from the real world through external stimulation and input can be a way to decompress, or it can be placing a Band-Aid over the overwhelm we feel. I recommend finding a balance between consumption and creation, as well as a balance between giving and receiving.

Limiting External Inputs

The cycle of stimulation, overwhelm, and anxiety can become toxic. It begins with too much input, leading to feelings of exhaustion and unfulfillment, which then drive us to seek even more stimulation or make impulsive choices. It's a loop many of us have found ourselves in at one point or another.

Now, let's shift our focus to material stimulation. I first grasped this concept after my partner and I had our son, Bodhi. As a new mom, I was immediately immersed in a world of flashing lights, loud toys, and endless distractions. It all felt like too much. So when Bodhi was born, I had intentional conversations with my partner, family, and friends about prioritizing low-stimulation environments. Open-ended play, wooden toys, and natural exploration became the focus. I'm not a strict mom; he watches TV occasionally, but I stick to slow-paced programs and limit screen time. I also rotate his toys, keeping only a few out at a time while storing the rest, so he has variety without excess. I will admit I'm a sucker for impulse buys at Target—it's something I'm working on. The point is, I'm not perfect, but I've become more conscious of how material stimulation affects all of us.

When Bodhi was around six months old, we went over

to the home of a mom-friend who had a little boy around the same age. Her living room was filled to the brim with rolling, flashing, loud toys. Bodhi was sitting there for at least twenty minutes just completely overwhelmed. The mom kept handing Bodhi a new flashing toy, and each time he gave me a worried look. He eventually found blocks that were familiar to him and played with those.

The stark contrast of environments between the friend's house and ours made something extremely clear to me: **The more stuff we have around us, the more overwhelmed we become.** In fact, there have been multiple empirical studies conducted that conclude materialism has a direct and profound impact on our overall psychological well-being. And children in general are more sensitive to their environments, which means we should be even more aware of their external world. When we overexpose them to too much stimulation, they become used to it and then expect it. And, of course, when that level of stimulation isn't available to that child, they react negatively. These days so many toys and products are designed to "keep kids engaged." But engaged in what, exactly? Keeping their attention? Preventing boredom? It makes me wonder: Are we projecting our own addiction to stimulation onto our children? Who decided that a two-year-old needs an iPad just to make it through a trip to the grocery store? Is it really for the child, or is it because they've become so accustomed to external stimuli that, without it, they feel anxious? Or perhaps it happens because the parents need a break? What I've observed in public spaces is even more concerning. Families sit together at restaurants, yet no one is speaking or even making eye contact; everyone is glued to a device, children included, often with headphones on. It's as if we've forgotten how to simply exist without constant input. And the more I pay attention, the more I realize just how deeply ingrained this cycle of overstimulation has become in our society. All of this leads to long-term concerns and implications for future generations.

As adults, we are constantly surrounded by stimulation, especially because technology (particularly our smartphones) often plays a dominant role in our lives. When was the last time you truly engaged with your five senses, one at a time? When was the last time you paused to take in a scent simply for the experience of smelling it? Or tasted something without simultaneously talking, listening, or watching a screen? When was the last time you did absolutely nothing, not even thinking, just to be? To be clear, I'm not against material things. I use my phone every day, like everyone else. The key is awareness, recognizing the ways in which constant stimulation shapes our experience and, ultimately, impacts our mental and emotional health.

So what do I suggest? Limit your material world. We are physical beings, which means it's necessary to own physical things to help us do basic tasks—like eating on a plate with a fork and knife, for instance. But we have a tendency to surround ourselves with stuff we don't need and overbuy, especially when something is cheap. For example, I have about ten pairs of sunglasses. Each pair I buy costs about ten bucks. Do I *need* ten pairs of sunglasses? No, of course not—not to mention, the momentary anxiety I feel when I open a drawer full of them and can't pick which ones best go with that day's outfit. My partner, on the other hand, has one pair of one-hundred-dollar sunglasses, which she's had for about five years now. She keeps them clean and safe and never has to worry about which ones go with her outfit—she has one pair. Because I have the mentality that my sunglasses are affordable and cheap, I do not value them the same. I buy extra pairs I don't wear or leave them places never to see them again. I'm actually spending more time, money, and energy keeping up with all my pairs of sunglasses.

At a certain point, collecting more stuff is detrimental to you rather than beneficial. **The mental process around consuming more stuff is just as addictive, if not more addictive, than the thing itself.** I opened an Amazon package the other day and felt like it was Christmas, only to have that feeling evaporate once I had that dish towel I'd bought in my hands.

Ask yourself: What is it for you? What material possessions in your life are extra or unnecessary? For some people it's shoes, makeup, clothing, or even food. Do you have a random CD collection you just can't let go of? Maybe you collect magnets from the countries you've visited. It's okay to indulge in some extra material things that bring you joy, such as the vast crystal collection I have. But at the rate at which we are shopping, spending, and consuming, our sense of ease is bound to be thrown off with feelings of overwhelm. Part of me knows that society will become so overwhelmed with material stuff that eventually we are *all* going to yearn for a more simplified and focused way of living.

You do not need to fill every corner of your space with stuff. It will stress you out even if you aren't fully aware of it. So save yourself the time, money, energy, and anxiety by limiting what you buy and clearing out what you have. One of the things I've been trying to implement in my own life is buying quality things that last a long time, rather than cheaper alternatives that have to be replaced every year. This fosters a deeper awareness, not just of the item's quality, but also of its origin, the materials used, and its overall impact on the world. I also go through all my cupboards and drawers and closets every few months, and go through my entire fridge and freezer every week before I go grocery shopping. A good rule of thumb for anything is: If you haven't used it within the past six months, you most likely don't need it. (An obvious exception to that rule is seasonal materials like winter clothing.) Another way to deep dive and clear out your materials is asking yourself, "Does this item bring me joy?" If you say "one day it will" or the answer is no, get rid of it. You can pass something along, donate it, or sell it before thinking of just throwing it out. Likewise, and I hate saying it, if you are holding on to stuff from your parents or grandparents, or your childhood, and it doesn't bring you joy, let it go. You will be better off for it. **By pausing to consciously consider our consumption choices, rather than acting on autopilot, we make more intentional and responsible decisions that benefit both ourselves and the world around us.**

Try to include a deep cleaning and organization every few months. It will drastically improve your anxiety levels. Don't try to tackle the whole house at once; start small with just a drawer or closet so that managing your physical space isn't as overwhelming. Just like when we try to tackle the anxiety in our mind, by breaking it down and focusing on the past, present, and future, it becomes easier and easier to navigate. I heard a saying once that goes **"a cluttered home is a cluttered**

mind," and it really rings true for my own life. Speaking of minds, let's now turn our attention to the internal world and how overstimulating your mind can lead to more anxiety.

The Comfort Trap: Why Avoiding Discomfort Fuels Anxiety

Our brains are wired for pattern recognition. They thrive on predictability because it allows us to respond efficiently to familiar situations. The more we repeat certain actions and responses, the stronger the neural pathways get. This process ensures that familiar experiences require less conscious effort over time. For example, when you first learn to drive, every movement requires focus, checking mirrors, positioning your hands, and gauging your speed. But with repetition, these actions become second nature. Eventually, you can drive while thinking about your grocery list or singing along to a song without actively focusing on each step. This efficiency is useful in many aspects of life, but when it comes to emotional and behavioral responses, it can keep us stuck in patterns that no longer serve us.

Many people structure their lives to maintain this sense of familiarity, often without realizing it. In the Western world, much of our daily existence revolves around seeking comfort and minimizing discomfort. We upgrade our technology to make life easier, adjust our environments to feel more at ease, and avoid situations that might challenge us. We eat at the same restaurants, take the same routes to work, and socialize with the same people. While comfort and routine provide stability, they can also create complacency and reinforce a fear of the unknown. **Over time, avoiding discomfort becomes a habit, one that strengthens neural pathways associated with resistance to change.**

The problem is that life *is* unpredictable. When we become too reliant on comfort and routine, any deviation from the expected outcomes can trigger anxiety. This is why change, whether it's a new job, a move, or even a minor disruption in our plans, often feels overwhelming and could trigger anxiety. **The brain perceives it as a potential threat simply because it's unfamiliar.** By constantly choosing the familiar, we unknowingly reinforce the belief that the unknown is dangerous. Instead of building resilience, we condition ourselves to fear change. But what if, instead of avoiding discomfort, we leaned into it? What if we treated uncertainty as an opportunity for growth rather than something to fear?

Breaking free from this cycle doesn't mean eliminating comfort altogether; it means finding a balance. When we intentionally step outside our comfort zones, even in small ways, we teach our brains that uncertainty isn't something to be avoided; it's something we are capable of handling. The more we practice embracing change, the more adaptable and, ultimately, less anxious we become.

New Actions: Rewiring Your Brain for Change

This is a technique I've taught many clients over the years and still apply in my own life today. It aligns perfectly with the "getting uncomfortable" section because stepping into new actions naturally pushes us outside our comfort zones, forcing us to confront the internal safety mechanisms that resist change. By intentionally making unexpected choices, we activate a heightened sense of awareness while simultaneously challenging the brain's established patterns. This process disrupts our autopilot mode, encouraging new neural pathways to form and making us more adaptable to change.

Do something completely random, right now.

Seriously, don't just read this, do it. Pick an action that feels completely out of the ordinary for you. For example, as I'm writing this, I just grabbed a pen and threw it across the room. Then I took my gum out of my mouth and stuck it to the back of my hand. Neither of these actions are things I would normally do, and that's the point. At that moment, my brain had no automatic response. It was caught off guard, unsure of how to react. But by doing something unexpected, I just created a new neural pathway, one that tells my brain that **random and unfamiliar things can happen, and that's okay.**

Back when I was deep into understanding mental reprogramming, I used to randomly clap my hands at different intervals just to disrupt my daily expectations. It sounds ridiculous, and honestly, it kind of was, but these small, spontaneous changes had a massive impact on my anxiety. They trained my brain to expect the unexpected in a safe and playful way. Over time, this practice helped me handle major life changes, like buying a house or having a child, without spiraling into fear. **By conditioning my mind to accept minor uncertainties, I built resilience for handling bigger ones.**

Here's how you can apply this in your own life.

Start Small

Change something in your daily routine just for the sake of doing it differently:

- Make a paper airplane and throw it. Simple, random, and completely harmless.
- Switch up your meals. If you always have spaghetti on Wednesdays, make it on Friday. Or better yet, try a food you've never had before. Even if you hate it, you've still succeeded in breaking a pattern.
- Take a different route home. Walk or drive a different way to work and notice how your mind feels more engaged.
- Rearrange your furniture. You might love it, you might hate it, but you won't know until you try.

The more you introduce these small, harmless disruptions, the more your brain **adapts to change**. Over time, this rewiring teaches you that *the* unknown *is not* a threat; it's just something new. And when we stop fearing uncertainty, we stop letting anxiety control our decisions.

Cold Showers

Another technique for reprogramming our brains around discomfort is cold showers. There have been multiple studies investigating cold water and anxiety; findings show that we can improve our overall stress resilience by voluntarily facing discomfort, and that cold exposure can be linked to the release of endorphins, which can elevate mood and also help reduce anxiety.

I believe regular cold showers can help us experience discomfort in a way that gets us back into our body and helps us accept being uncomfortable in the future. From my own experience, it not only builds that stress resilience, but it makes you really appreciate warm water when you have it. The more you push yourself into uncomfortable situations (in a safe way), the easier it will be to navigate the unknown challenges of the future. This not only builds confidence and trust between you and the outside world, it also builds a deep foundation of self-worth along with it.

The Foundation of Self-Care

If you're constantly exhausted, running on caffeine and stress, skipping meals, or pushing through burnout, it doesn't matter how much inner work you do, your body simply won't have the resources to support you. Anxiety isn't just a mental or emotional experience; it's deeply connected to your physical well-being. And when your body is in survival mode, your mind will be too. Think about it: When you're overtired, everything feels heavier, harder, and more overwhelming. Small problems seem like massive roadblocks. The ability to separate your emotions from external energy, to regulate your thoughts, or to practice self-awareness is nearly impossible when your nervous system is already running on empty.

Anxiety thrives in a state of depletion. The more physically drained you are, the less capacity you have to process emotions, set boundaries, and regulate your energy. When your body isn't nourished or rested, your mind will look for something, anything, to explain why you feel so off. That's when anxious thoughts become louder, triggers feel more intense, and everything seems unmanageable. But when you prioritize your own well-being, something shifts. When you get enough sleep, when you eat foods that actually fuel you, when you create space for rest instead of constantly pushing through, it sends a message to your entire system:

"I am safe. I am supported. I am taking care of myself."

And that message is powerful. Self-care isn't just about checking off a to-do list; it's about building trust with yourself. Every time you meet your needs instead of ignoring them, you're reinforcing the belief that you've got your own back. You're proving to yourself that you are showing up for *you*, which creates an inner stability that anxiety can't shake as easily. On top of that, when you physically take care of yourself, you naturally neutralize some of the most common triggers that fuel present-moment anxiety. Hunger, exhaustion, and burnout all send stress signals to the brain, making it harder to regulate emotions and process external energy. When those stressors are minimized, you gain more space to navigate real emotional and energetic challenges, instead of being thrown into a spiral over something that could have been avoided with simple care.

At the end of the day, managing anxiety isn't just about mindset work or energetic practices. It starts with the basics, fueling your body, resting when you need to, and creating a foundation where your mind and emotions don't fight against you. The stronger your foundation, the more capacity you'll have to not only handle anxiety but to actually work with it as a tool.

Final Notes

Anxiety is a fickle thing. It affects everyone differently and comes from a multitude of places. As complex and overwhelming as it is to understand, it's an incredibly easy thing to catch. Anxiety is a signal telling us that something is wrong. However, our receiver is so inundated with external stimulation and past emotion, we aren't able to fully pick up on the initial signal; we ignore it until the symptoms become too loud. We aren't usually aware of where it came from and what it's trying to tell us. This confusion leads to the avalanche of symptoms our systems are trying to figure out.

As historic pack animals who hunted together, if someone else's alarm is going off, yours will too. In a world prompting us to engage through fear tactics, we are primed and ready to trigger that alarm at a moment's notice. Regardless of catching anxiety, regardless of the amount you consume or the external overwhelm you have in your orbit, you do have the power to stop it at its source.

By recognizing anxiety as it arises and challenging our automatic responses, we can break the cycle before it spirals. Instead of mindlessly consuming, we can prioritize creation to counterbalance our inputs with constructive outputs, and avoid surrounding ourselves with unnecessary "stuff" in the first place. Instead of trying to escape discomfort, we can retrain our minds to see change as something natural and beneficial, rather than a threat. A powerful way to do this is by making small, intentional changes in our daily routines. When we push ourselves to step outside our comfort zones, even in minor ways, we show our brains that uncertainty isn't dangerous. Small shifts help reprogram your autopilot and make you more adaptable to the unknown. To take it even further, you can introduce physical discomfort, like cold showers, to reinforce your ability to handle uncertainty. **The more we expose ourselves to safe but uncomfortable experiences, the more we teach our nervous system that we don't need to react with fear.** This process builds resilience, strengthens our ability to navigate stress, and ultimately reduces anxiety in the long run. Prioritizing self-care is also key. When we are physically and emotionally depleted, anxiety becomes even harder to manage. By getting enough sleep, nourishing our bodies, and creating space for rest, we reinforce an internal sense of stability that makes it easier to handle life's unpredictability.

Stepping into discomfort, rewiring your automatic responses, and taking care of yourself are the real tools for navigating anxiety in the present and for the future. You've got this, anxiety ally. I'm right here with you!

Key Chapter Takeaways

- Conscious consumption versus creation: Anxiety increases when we input more than we output.
- You can decrease overwhelm by decluttering and creating intentional habits.
- Getting uncomfortable in a safe way reprograms

your autopilot system into understanding that change and the unknown isn't something to be feared, but instead, something to enjoy.

Key Action Steps

- Declutter one small space in your home (physical clutter = mental clutter).
- Change up your routine by choosing something different or random in the moment.
- Allow yourself to get uncomfortable more often. It might be a conversation you would have avoided or opting for that cold shower to kick off your day.

Client Case Study
Sarah: Breaking Free

Sarah was drowning in overwhelm. When I met her, she was a single mom and a full-time administrative assistant, which meant her days were spent juggling, fixing, responding, and handling everything for everyone else. She barely had time to breathe, let alone process her emotions. During one of our first sessions, I asked her point-blank, "When do you have time for yourself?"

Sarah laughed out loud. "Time for myself? Between packing lunches, doing laundry, and just trying to show up for work on time, me-time isn't even possible."

I knew I needed to choose my next words carefully. "So when you do have a moment to sit in silence, maybe while driving to work or lying down at the end of the day, what comes up for you?"

Her face showed strong discomfort, maybe even anguish. "The silence is loud—it's full of guilt and regret and shame and blame, so I just tune it out. Sometimes it's easier to fall asleep with the TV on than it is listening to those thoughts." And this is what clued me in. I explained to her that anxiety isn't always dramatic. Sometimes it looks like perpetual exhaustion and the need to check out in order to rest.

It was clear to me that Sarah was absorbing

energy from everyone around her, her demanding job, the pressures of single parenting, even the emotions of the people she interacted with daily. And because she never released any of it, her nervous system did what it had to do to protect her: shut down. In order to shift her out of this survival mindset, I needed to guide her in a new direction.

I told her, "Do one small, unfamiliar thing each day."

Sarah immediately objected, "I don't have the time for a new morning routine." I reminded her that it wasn't about a new routine. It was about a new spark, something different to light her up. So she started that day. Instead of picking her daughter up and heading straight home, they went to the park instead. This didn't require extra energy on her part, but she noticed how her daughter lit up and even slept better after doing so. During another session, Sarah reported to me with a true, genuine smile on her face, "Last night, instead of turning on the TV, we built a fort out of the couch cushions and even ate our dinner in it. I don't remember the last time I laughed so hard." She also mentioned that she tried making green, healthy smoothies for them both. "It was disgusting, but we made a game out of who could drink it the fastest and both felt more energy after."

Each new choice was small, but slowly, she started weaving her life back together. With every new experience, it not only brought her closer to her daughter, but it brought her back into herself.

Within weeks, Sarah started *feeling* again. She was more present, more connected to her daughter, more alive. Her anxiety didn't push her into disconnecting anymore. She wasn't just surviving the day; she was living it.

If you're caught in a cycle of avoiding, numbing, or just going through the motions, ask yourself, "What small shift can I make today?" Sometimes, it's not about changing everything; it's about changing one thing that sparks something inside you again.

Chapter 5

Anxiety Alchemy: Rewriting the Future

Hey Anxiety Ally,

Have you ever been lying in bed, staring at the ceiling, as your mind takes you on a never-ending ride through future what-ifs? Maybe you've got a friend's birthday party coming up, and you find yourself wondering, What will I wear? Who's going to be there? Will I even know enough people to feel comfortable? *Or perhaps it's something a little more serious, like a new dog sitter coming over for the first time. Will they take good care of your pup? What if something terrible happens, like your dog escaping the leash and running off?*

The possibilities are endless, and the thoughts? Relentless. It's like your brain is trying to map out every scenario, big or small, to make sure you're prepared for everything. But instead of feeling in control, you end up trapped in a loop of overthinking, unable to stop.

If you're anything like me, you've probably tried to escape this spiral by distracting yourself. Maybe you open TikTok, hoping that a couple of funny videos will drown out the noise. And you know what? It works, for a little while. But inevitably, the next worry sneaks in, and before you know it, you're back in the loop, replaying the same exhausting cycle.

If this sounds familiar, then this chapter is for you. We're about to dive into the wild world of future anxiety, those thoughts that pull you out of the present and into a tangled mess of infinite what-ifs. The exciting part is that your anxiety isn't your enemy; it can actually be a tool.

This isn't about silencing your mind or avoiding your thoughts. It's about learning to work with your anxiety, channel it into something productive, and navigate your life with clarity and purpose. You're not powerless in the face of your worries. You're powerful, and this chapter is going to show you just how much.

Let's dive in and start turning those anxious "what-ifs" into a confident "I've got this." You're ready for this next step—let's go!

What Is Future Anxiety?

When your spidey sense alert goes off, your mind gets focused on what it perceives as the *biggest* threat. So, believe it or not, having anxious thoughts about the future can be a good sign. It's often a clear indication that you've done a fair amount of work on yourself. You see, if you still needed to heal the past, your anxious thoughts would be focused on the past. When you've done work on healing trauma and unresolved emotions, your mind hyper-focuses on the future as the cause of the alarm trigger instead. (Just because your mind worries about the future doesn't mean you have healed *all* of the past, but it's a good indication you are making big strides.) However, the main issue persists: Your alarm bells are ringing, and your mind is attempting to justify this signal by finding something to blame.

Future anxiety is the emotional discomfort, stress, or fear experienced when our thoughts become preoccupied with uncertain events that have not yet taken place. It arises from imagining negative outcomes, which often leads to a sense of helplessness or loss of control. Future anxiety manifests as excessive worry, apprehension, or unease about what might happen, which then interferes with our sense of calm. In other words, future anxiety pulls our mental and emotional focus away from the present moment into hypotheticals—usually worst-case scenarios. This creates unnecessary stress because our minds perceive potential threats that we currently have no immediate control over. Common examples of future anxiety include worries about financial security, career success, relationships, health concerns, or global and societal issues. The *uncertainty* about what will—or could—happen in the future tends to magnify anxiety and intensify our emotional reaction.

It's important to recognize that future anxiety is driven primarily by *perception* rather than *reality*. Our imagination inflates potential risks, often blowing them out of proportion, creating more emotional distress. Our minds only ever land on these imaginary fears because they are trying to alert us to something.

Conventional therapy methods like mindfulness will have you refocus on the present moment when one of these episodes arise. Although it's important to regain your perspective by bringing your awareness into the present, this technique won't end the anxiety for good. It will only stop it in the moment. So what *will* end future anxiety for good? Trust. **Creating an ongoing sense of trust within yourself helps you to feel like no matter what life throws at you, you can manage.**

Creating this trust takes time. We aren't just trying to solve the symptoms; we are trying to reprogram your brain so that they don't arise in the first place. Reprogramming takes time, dedication, and, most of all, *awareness*. And in order to have full awareness, we must prioritize *ourselves* over others and over external factors in life that we can't control.

This chapter contains the core of my anxiety solutions. So don't feel like you need to just apply them to your future anxieties. Applying them to all aspects of your life will greatly benefit your overall well-being and freedom.

Taking Your Power Back from Future Anxiety

So far, we've covered ways to handle anxiety caused by past and present situations. Now it's time to deal with future anxiety, not just to manage it, but also to use what we've learned to improve our lives. I want to introduce you to my main anxiety strategy. I call it ReNU for short, and it stands for

"Recognize, Neutralize, and Utilize." With regular practice and application, this strategy not only stops anxiety spirals in their tracks, it will also help you sustainably end the cycle of anxiety altogether.

Recognize

One of the most powerful things we can do when dealing with anxiety is **recognize when we're experiencing it.** Just noticing our anxious state is already a huge accomplishment. Anxiety, as uncomfortable as it feels, actually has a unique advantage: **It makes us hyperaware.** Much like physical pain, anxiety demands our immediate attention and pulls us deep into our own minds through its discomfort.

When you're working on healing anxiety, it's crucial to catch yourself in the very moment anxiety strikes. This can be challenging, especially with future-focused anxiety, because our minds love to conjure up vivid worst-case scenarios. These imaginary situations can feel incredibly real since they trigger a powerful emotional response in our bodies. **Research shows that our brains can't tell the difference between something that's actually happening and something we're just imagining.** A notable study from University College London (UCL) explored how vividly imagined experiences can blur the line between imagination and reality. Participants were asked to imagine visual patterns, such as alternating black and white lines, while their brain activity was monitored. The findings revealed that the brain encodes the vividness of both real and imagined stimuli in a similar manner, which can lead to confusion between actual perception and imagination. What this means is that anxious thoughts can feel just as real as lived experiences.

Typically, when future anxiety arises, our attention naturally shifts to the emotional drama of these imagined scenarios, rather than the anxiety itself. Here's the subtle yet transformative shift you can make: Instead of getting caught up in the story your mind is creating, gently redirect your awareness back to the feeling of anxiety itself—the tightness, the racing heartbeat, the tension. By simply observing the anxiety as a present-moment experience rather than engaging with anxious thoughts about the future, you effectively interrupt the cycle. This small change in awareness can significantly shift a limiting, stressful mental state into one of clarity, freedom, and calm.

It's important to understand that the entire cycle of anxiety, from the initial spidey sense alert to the physical and emotional symptoms that follow, is simply a mechanism designed to get your attention. Your body and mind are not working against you. They are trying to signal that something feels off, even if you can't immediately identify what it is. Most of us experience anxiety as a reaction to these signals rather than a message to be observed. When we don't recognize the alert early on, our subconscious ramps up the volume, escalating symptoms in order to force us to pay attention. The longer we ignore or resist these signals, the louder they become. This is why anxiety often feels like it spirals out of control; the body is desperately trying to be heard.

If you start the cycle with full awareness and recognition, the symptoms no longer need to "yell" to get your

attention. The moment you acknowledge the initial alert, without fear, judgment, or immediate action, you interrupt the entire chain reaction. Instead of being caught off guard and thrown into a spiral, you create space to respond *intentionally* rather than reacting impulsively. Think of it like an alarm clock. If you wake up at the first sound, there's no need for it to keep blaring, creating a sense of panic in us. Anxiety works the same way. When you tune in early, acknowledging, observing, and staying present, you take back control of your nervous system. Instead of letting anxiety dictate your experience, you shift into a state of *conscious navigation.*

One of the easiest ways to bring recognition to your initial anxiety triggers is to get curious about it. Curiosity will open your mind and help you to observe the symptoms and triggers rather than fear them and respond with the fight, flight, or freeze mechanisms. Here are two questions you can ask to help support your recognition and curiosity.

What is my body trying to tell me right now?

Instead of reacting to the physical discomfort, approach it with curiosity. Pay attention to signs like a racing heart, sweating, tight chest, or restlessness. By observing the sensations in our body, we are able to ground back into the present moment and switch our attention from our racing minds to something more tangible. Typically, when we begin to feel anxiety symptoms, we try to mask or mitigate them by distracting ourselves from them. By bringing your awareness to the sensations, you can begin changing your response to them from fear to curiosity.

What thoughts are looping in my mind; what are they focused on?

Asking this question helps you recognize repetitive or negative thought patterns. Instead of getting caught up in the emotional response to your thoughts, this shifts you into a state of curiosity, allowing you to *observe* anxiety rather than fear it. When you approach your thoughts with curiosity instead of resistance, you create space to learn from them rather than feeling like they are an enemy to battle. If you find it difficult to bring awareness to your thoughts in the moment, that's completely okay. Simply asking the question plants the seed of awareness, and over time, it becomes easier to recognize and understand your thought patterns.

By recognizing anxiety at its root, you can stop it from escalating before it ever takes over. That is the power of awareness. In fact, simply acknowledging its presence can significantly reduce its intensity. All anxiety truly wants is attention, and recognition can calm the nervous system and create distance between you and the anxious thoughts. This awareness helps to stop anxiety in the moment, offering immediate relief. However, recognition alone isn't enough to prevent anxiety from returning. If we want to create long-term change, we must go deeper. This brings us to the second step of ReNU: neutralize.

Neutralize

Anxiety isn't something we can simply eliminate; it's something we must reprogram. The mind has been conditioned to respond to uncertainty with fear, and these responses have been reinforced over time, making them automatic. Before we can override these deeply ingrained mental pathways, we must first *neutralize* them.

Neutrality: The state of complete balance and non-attachment to polarizing energies. It's the ability to observe reality without judgment, fear, or emotional reactivity, allowing you to remain centered no matter what external chaos unfolds.

Neutrality is the bridge between awareness and transformation. Without it, we remain stuck in the cycle, recognizing anxiety but still reacting to it as a threat. Neutralizing our automatic responses allows us to shift from reacting with fear to responding with clarity. Through years of working with clients, and my own experiences of trial and error, I've identified two key ways to neutralize unwanted thoughts and anxious responses:

1. **Safety:** Reassuring the nervous system that you are not in danger, so the anxiety cycle no longer needs to escalate.
2. **Observation:** Learning to witness anxious thoughts without emotional attachment, so they lose their power over you.

In the following sections, I'll break down these two techniques in depth. When used together, they form the foundation for rewiring your brain's relationship with anxiety, transforming it from something that overwhelms you into something you can navigate with confidence.

Safety

Historically, our survival depended on responding to threats the moment our instincts were triggered. But today, our spidey sense alarm is constantly overstimulated by non-life-threatening triggers. Instead of helping us survive, it's limiting our ability to fully live. And the real issue, as I've stated before, isn't the alert itself; it's *not knowing why the alert is there*.

At every level of our being, we fear the unknown. At a biological level, we fear the unknown because it could signal a hidden threat. Psychologically, we fear the unknown due to the possibility of failure, loss of control, or unexpected change. Past traumas and the need for predictability make uncertainty unsettling. At its core, all of these responses boil down to one thing: our need for *safety*. Our search for the cause of the spidey sense alert only amplifies our distress, reinforcing the belief that we are not safe. The truth, however, is that in most moments of anxiety, we *are not in real danger*.

To break this cycle, we must target the perceived lack of safety. The simplest and most effective way to do this is by actively reassuring our system of safety in the present moment. When you notice anxiety rising, pause and remind yourself:

"I am safe."

That's it, as simple as that. This affirmation interrupts the spiral by directly addressing the core fear, telling your subconscious mind that there is no immediate danger. To deepen this practice, add breathwork to reinforce the feeling of safety. The best breathing technique I've come across (and I've tried many!) is a method called "box breathing." Here's how to do it:

1. Inhale deeply for four seconds.
2. Hold your breath for four seconds.
3. Slowly exhale for four seconds.
4. Hold (empty lungs) for four seconds.

Box breathing directly engages your autonomic nervous system, especially the parasympathetic branch, which shifts the body out of the fight, flight, or freeze response and into the rest and digest response. It has been scientifically proven to help lower your heart rate, blood pressure, and cortisol levels. By consciously breathing in for four seconds, holding for four, exhaling for four, and holding again for four, you're signaling to your nervous system that you are safe. This calms the mind and reduces anxiety in the moment. It's a reset button for your body and your mind, especially in moments where fear or overwhelm takes over.

Repeat this at least three times while affirming in your mind, *I am safe*. This technique instantly reduces stress and signals to your brain that there is no real threat and it's time to calm down. It's a simple technique but an incredible hack for an overactive mind.

Remember that anxiety is inherently a safety mechanism. It's not trying to hurt you; it's trying to protect you. However, when we react with fear, we reinforce the belief that we *are* unsafe, causing anxiety to escalate. By consciously bringing ourselves into the present and affirming safety through engaging both our mind and body, we disrupt the cycle. We no longer need to identify a threat in order to feel better. **Instead, we remind our nervous system that we are *already* okay.**

You may need to repeat this process several times, especially if anxiety feels overwhelming, but with practice, this simple technique will retrain your brain to respond differently. And over time, your system will **learn that anxiety is not an enemy; it's just an alert that wants your attention.**

Observation

This next step can feel tricky, but it's powerful because it equips us with the essential tools we need for sustainable anxiety healing. Typically, when a worrying future scenario pops into our minds, we either get caught up in the emotional drama it triggers or we try to distract ourselves from it to avoid discomfort. Many traditional anxiety techniques suggest that we dismiss these thoughts, labeling them as "not real." However, doing that disconnects us from our intuition and internal warning system. If you genuinely want to transform anxiety into a superpower, you need to address and neutralize the underlying fear itself. Instead of avoiding that anxious thought, I want you to *observe* the imagined scenario fully, from beginning to end.

Objective Observation: Looking at a situation or thought without emotional judgment or reaction, enabling clarity and reducing anxiety.

For example, I once had a persistent fear of me or someone falling down the stairs while holding my newborn. This fear haunted me day and night, causing me to grip the railing tightly when I was carrying him, and micromanage anyone else who held my child near stairs. One night, I decided to let this imagined scenario play out completely in my mind. It was terrifying. I imagined falling, hearing my baby cry, rushing to the hospital . . . As I let myself replay this imagined event, each time ended slightly differently, sometimes with a concussion or even broken bones. As I vividly imagined this, my anxiety peaked, my body tensed, my heart raced, and my emotions spiraled into turmoil. Then I replayed the scene again, this time focusing on observing objectively with less emotional reaction. Any time a strong emotion came up, I would breathe deeply and remind myself that I was safe. My body still reacted, but less intensely. I noticed there was a clear peak of anxiety, followed by a de-escalation. The more I repeated this observation without emotionally reacting, the more I accepted the scenario as just another possibility rather than something terrifying.

To my amazement, the next day, my fear around the stairs completely disappeared. I stopped gripping the railing tightly and stopped micromanaging others. The possibility of falling didn't change—and it still existed—but by consciously experiencing it without emotional reaction, my mind no longer perceived it as an active threat needing my focus and attention. My anxiety around the situation was neutralized.

Here's exactly how you can apply this technique when anxiety loops through your mind:

1. **Deep Breathing:** Begin with the box breathing technique and reminder of safety we covered earlier in this chapter. (Calm your nervous system with slow, intentional breaths: Inhale for four seconds, hold for four, exhale for four, and hold again for another four. Remember, 4-4-4-4.)
2. **Reassure Yourself of Safety:** Remind yourself that you are safe. This helps you step out of feeling immersed in the scenario, allowing you to observe it instead.
3. **Observe the Imagined Scenario:** Pick one recurring anxious thought and mentally play it out from start to finish. Initially, you will experience intense anxiety symptoms, and your initial instinct will be to avoid it.
4. **Repeat Your Safety Reminder:** Remind yourself again that you are safe, and continue deep breathing.
5. **Replay Until Neutralized:** Keep replaying the scenario until your emotional reaction significantly diminishes or disappears completely. Once the scenario no longer triggers negative emotions, you've successfully neutralized it!

This approach is similar to how we heal past traumas. We're not changing the events themselves, or potential future events, but by consciously observing and accepting them, **we reclaim our emotional power.** This technique doesn't disconnect you emotionally; it allows you to move safely and consciously through difficult emotions. Interestingly, I find that stress dreams can function similarly, providing a safe environment for your mind to process uncomfortable scenarios so they no longer cause distress during your waking life. Our minds naturally love observing and solving problems. When we allow ourselves to feel anxiety-provoking scenarios, we reassure our subconscious that these scenarios aren't hidden threats; **they're experiences we're equipped to handle.** By consciously choosing to feel and observe anxiety, we remove the power it has over us, and our minds no longer see it as something needing resolution.

Utilize

When we reach the point of neutralizing anxiety, we unlock something incredibly valuable: a conscious space of clarity and choice. This moment is powerful because, for once, we are not reacting impulsively to anxiety; we are fully present and in control. Most people seek immediate relief from anxiety through medication, distractions, or self-soothing with food and other comforts. While these coping mechanisms can offer temporary ease, they skip over the opportunity that anxiety has created: a rare moment of heightened awareness. Once the anxiety fades, we tend to move on without reflecting on what just happened or how we could use that experience to our advantage. But this space is a gift. It's a pause, a break from autopilot mode, where you have the freedom to choose your next move consciously. Instead of letting the moment pass, why not utilize it for something meaningful?

Check In

One of the ways you can utilize this conscious moment is to check in with yourself. Create an open dialogue about your day, your interactions, or your emotions. Use it as a time to internally journal to yourself. The more we talk consciously to ourselves, the more trust we build within ourselves. Everyone needs to be heard, and that includes you! This new trust will empower you to seek help from *yourself* rather than external forces. Just like checking up on an old friend, you deserve that too.

Bring Gratitude

Utilize this moment of awareness to focus on something in your life you feel grateful for. Is it your pet or your partner? Is it your ability to show up for yourself? What in your life brings you joy and a feeling of abundance? Maybe it's the flowers blooming in your neighborhood or a pantry full of food. It's easy to find appreciation, but not always easy to find the time to do it. Gratitude overall will raise your energy levels, which will also help you lessen the severity and sustainability of anxiety. The more gratitude, the better!

Manifest Something

If you're really feeling present and aligned after recognizing the anxiety, and then neutralizing it through observation and safety, poke around to see if there is anything you are wanting to manifest. Maybe it's a new job or just more financial freedom. No matter what it is, utilize this moment of awareness to focus on the reality where you *already* have the things you desire. What would it look like to have your dream house? What would it feel like to do something that is deeply fulfilling? There is no limit to what you can create, so go for it!

If you are new to manifestation, know that something

only gets manifested if you perceive yourself as already having it. So instead of focusing on what you want in the future, such as saying, "I will be anxiety free," say instead, "I am anxiety free," even if you don't fully believe it. Words are powerful, and by always placing our intentions into the future, they will remain there. It's important to bring your focus and desires into the now in order to expedite their creation.

By using this moment intentionally, you **retrain your brain to associate anxiety with *growth*, not just relief.** You shift from reacting to anxiety to *learning from it.* The more you practice utilizing this space, the more empowered you become, not only in managing anxiety but in utilizing it as a superpower.

In a world that constantly demands our attention, these moments of conscious awareness are rare. So the next time you recognize and neutralize your anxiety, don't just move on. Pause, breathe, and make the most of the space you've created.

Vibrational Navigation

Many years ago, I felt completely overwhelmed and helpless. It seemed like life was hitting me from every direction, from paying bills, answering emails, to helping others and trying to heal my own trauma. At any given moment, my body was busy doing one thing, while my mind was juggling three others. I'd be answering an email, but already worrying about the next meeting I had to join. It was exhausting.

On top of an already busy life, I started to open up my spiritual gifts again. Suddenly, I could sense the deeper energetic connections and layers beyond the physical world around me. These extra layers became too much to handle. I was no longer just managing the daily grind. I was also navigating all these unseen energies and subtle emotional threads. It felt like I was living in two worlds at once, and that constant balancing act created even more anxiety. At one point, I seriously considered going back to my blissful ignorance. Maybe if I just focused on making money, paying my bills, and getting through the day without worrying about anything deeper, life would feel simpler. Well, I tried it, and honestly, it made me miserable. Limiting myself to the physical world alone was easy, but it left me feeling disconnected and empty. **I realized the solution wasn't to ignore these deeper insights; it was to learn how to handle them properly.**

That's when I developed a concept called "Vibrational Navigation," or VN for short. Vibrational Navigation is the ability to consciously connect or disconnect from the world around us whenever we choose. The reality is, we're already connecting and disconnecting from things all the time; we just usually do it unconsciously. The difference now is becoming *aware* of this choice and making it *intentional.*

Vibrational Navigation (VN): Consciously choosing when and how deeply you connect or disconnect emotionally and energetically with your surroundings.

Think of making daily choices on autopilot mode. Our biology, society, and past traumas have created this subconscious autopilot system, a default response where we mentally check out, and our preprogramming turns on. When we're familiar with an experience or don't really care to engage with it fully, we simply drift away mentally and let autopilot take over. Imagine being stuck in traffic (something many of us know all too well). You have two main choices: You can either disconnect, zone out, and feel helpless, or you can engage negatively, becoming frustrated and angry about the wasted time. Usually, this decision happens without us even noticing. But our reactions can vary dramatically, depending on our physical and emotional state. If we're hungry, tired, or stressed, our reactions tend to be stronger because our body's natural flight, flight, or freeze response kicks in. What if in the moment of being stuck in traffic you were able to observe your current state? What happens if, instead of automatically reacting to the situation at hand, you observe it, and then choose how to respond to it? **In that split second of stepping back to observe and then choose, we change everything about who we are and how we respond to the world.** Learning how to consciously connect and disconnect from the world around you is the secret to mastering your reality and your anxiety. So, how do you actually do this?

Step 1: Awareness

The first and most important step is awareness. The only difference between regular connecting and disconnecting (that autopilot mode) and true Vibrational Navigation is becoming *conscious* of your choices. Through consistently practicing awareness, you teach your subconscious mind to step back so you can take the lead in the present moment. This process builds a sense of independence, safety, and self-worth, reducing anxiety in the long run. The problem is that being "more aware" is much harder than it sounds. Our lives are busy, our minds are constantly occupied, and our daily routines make it tough to pause and reflect. Anxiety and physical discomfort naturally pull us into awareness, but these are often uncomfortable reminders. To start building this skill without discomfort, you can use a simple trick: setting an alarm on your phone.

Set an alarm on your phone once or even three times a day for twenty-one days (studies suggest this is the amount of time needed to form a new habit). When the alarm goes off, pause and check in with yourself. Notice how you feel physically and emotionally in the moment. Are you hungry, tired, anxious, hot, or cold? Maybe you're happy, sad, or stressed. Just noticing your current state sends a powerful message to your subconscious mind: **that you're paying attention to the present moment**. In that moment, you are telling your autopilot to step back and let you take the lead.

At the end of this book, you will find a twenty-one-day anxiety survival guide. It incorporates everything covered in the book, including this alarm, into practical day-to-day activities.

Remember that when the alarm goes off, you're not trying to fix or judge anything in that moment; you're just acknowledging what's there. Giving yourself these brief moments of intentional awareness throughout the day will dramatically ease anxiety and improve your ability to navigate both your physical and energetic worlds. With practice, you'll find it easier to connect to the energy around you, experience lucid dreams, or even explore deeper spiritual realms, all through simply choosing to stay consciously aware. More awareness in and of itself creates a profound sense of trust in yourself and your own ability to navigate the world around you. **You are no longer a victim of circumstance but rather start the journey of taking responsibility for your actions, because you showed up presently to make them.**

Step 2: To Connect or Disconnect?

After you have created more awareness in your life, you then have to take the next step. You have a choice here: to connect or disconnect.

Connection

Connection is a simple yet powerful concept. When you watch a movie and cry because something tragic occurs, you're experiencing a connection to that moment. Similarly, if I ask you to imagine slamming your fingers in a door and you feel a visceral reaction, you're clearly connected and reacting to that thought. As I mentioned earlier in the book, overstimulation from our external and internal worlds creates so many connections that it becomes a tangled web we struggle to unravel. Eventually, we reach a point of saturation, like the oversaturated sponge, unable to absorb more, causing us to disconnect entirely and exist in a perpetual state of fuzziness.

There are two forms of connection: physical and nonphysical. As with real and imagined experiences, our brains typically don't differentiate between them, which is why they can both trigger anxiety. To connect consciously with either, we first need to pause, create a moment of awareness, and then actively choose to connect. Physical connections can be established easily through our five senses. For example, if I want to consciously connect with my cup of coffee, I might look at it, noticing its muddy brown color. I pick it up, smell its acidic aroma, and taste it, only to realize it's cold and no longer appealing. This observation sparks curiosity—why would I choose to drink something I don't truly enjoy? Perhaps it's an automatic habit or a lack of mindfulness about alternative choices. While this observation isn't the primary point of this section, it illustrates the profound impact conscious awareness can have on our everyday choices.

Conscious Connection: Deliberately engaging your attention and senses with something in your environment, physically or energetically.

But how do I connect energetically with my cup of coffee? It's just an inanimate object, so how is this done? We are energetic beings, constantly interacting with the world both through our five physical senses *and* through our sixth sense, our intuition. The easiest way to tap in to this extrasensory ability is to pay attention to our emotional responses. So I'm going to tune in to my coffee again, this time through my emotions. "How do I *feel* about this cold cup of coffee right now?" Honestly, indifferent. Maybe an hour ago, when hot and paired with a biscotti, it brought me joy; now it just feels cold, sad, and stale. By consciously connecting with our surroundings through both a physical and an emotional lens, we become aware of our intrinsic responses. Typically, these connections occur without our conscious knowledge, leaving us unaware of how our bodies and minds are responding to the external world. Let's add a practical step to the phone alarm system you've set up:

1. The alarm goes off.
2. You pause and check in with yourself.
3. You choose something in your immediate environment and consciously connect with it, engaging both your physical senses and emotional responses.

I highly recommend starting with simple, everyday aspects of life. Physical connections are straightforward since they are the primary focus of our daily experience. Energetic or emotional connections, however, can quickly become complicated and overwhelming, which is precisely why our brains often generate anxiety around them. For instance, imagine you have an elderly dog nearing the end of their life. When your awareness alarm prompts you to consciously connect, you choose to connect with them. You immediately notice an unpleasant smell coming from them. You go to pet them and can feel the rough and aged texture of their fur.

Moving to your emotions, you're flooded with joyful memories of adventures shared, quickly followed by sadness as you acknowledge their current pain and fragility. Such complex connections, without mastering Vibrational Navigation first, can easily spiral you into anxiety. Thus, when practicing conscious connection and VN, start simple and then gradually engage with more complex aspects of your reality.

By overriding our autopilot tendencies with conscious choices, we build trust in ourselves and our ability to navigate life intentionally. This intentional awareness helps calm our spidey sense alerts, as we begin to genuinely listen to and honor our subtle inner cues.

Disconnection

While it's essential to consciously connect with aspects of your life, it's equally important to consciously disconnect. As I've previously mentioned, when we feel anxious or overwhelmed, our minds naturally disconnect or disassociate to preserve energy and ensure our safety. This automatic response is a protection mechanism that serves us, initially. However, when left unchecked, these automatic disconnections lead to chronic anxiety over time. Stress serves as a powerful indicator of our overall well-being, and suppressed emotions inevitably burden our physical and emotional systems, causing the oversaturated sponge syndrome. We often unconsciously cope with stress by using social media, snack foods, or online shopping as a means of disconnecting. While these may temporarily relieve the overwhelm, they don't address the root issues and can eventually contribute to more stress. The key to effective disconnection lies in *intentionality.*

By consciously disconnecting from overwhelming situations, you regain control.

Conscious Disconnection: Intentionally disengaging your emotional or physical attention from a situation, thought, or person to regain mental clarity.

For example, if your whole house feels like an overwhelming mess, consciously disconnecting from that sense of overwhelm and instead focusing your attention on just one manageable space, like the kitchen, can significantly reduce anxiety and make tasks feel more achievable. Mastering conscious disconnection isn't about substituting one connection for another; that's like quitting smoking only to become addicted to chewing gum. **The goal is genuine detachment, not replacement.** To achieve this, you need a consistent anchor, and your breath serves as the perfect constant. When you're awake at 3 AM, overly connected to anxiety about possible future scenarios, consciously reconnecting with your breath helps ground you in reality, reminding you that the threat isn't present in that exact moment.

Here's a simple approach for conscious disconnection:

1. **Awareness:** Recognize when you're overly connected to something that's causing anxiety or stress.
2. **Refocus with Breath:** Practice the box breathing technique (page 105). This method helps break the emotional ties causing overwhelm, anchoring you firmly in the present.

Your breath is free from sensory distractions and emotional complexities, reminding you of the control you have over your reality. It's not external circumstances like your boss, your in-laws, or finances creating your reality; it's you.

If breath-focused techniques are challenging for you, I recommend incorporating another powerful method I mentioned earlier in the book: cord cutting (page 63). Remember that every interaction we have creates energetic connections, or cords. Weak cords—like the example of the interaction with the cup of coffee—will dissipate naturally, but intense emotional attachments form stronger ones that can hang around. Visualizing yourself cutting these cords helps neutralize their impact. This isn't a onetime action; repeated cord cutting maintains healthy boundaries and declutters your mind. Revisit page 62 if you need a refresher on how to clear energy cords.

When faced with particularly strong emotional attachments, actively disconnecting from these worries by anchoring into your breath or cord cutting and bringing awareness back to the present moment will help exponentially. When I find my mind rolling around future scenarios when I'm trying to get some sleep, I recognize what's happening and then cut the cord between the thought and myself. Whenever I do this, I feel immediately at ease. By consciously disconnecting, you neutralize anxieties, regaining clarity and power over your emotional state. After regularly practicing conscious disconnection, you'll notice greater mental clarity, reduced anxiety, increased motivation, and more energy overall. Your system will no longer be overwhelmed by external stresses. You'll be clearer, calmer, and more energized, giving you space to fully engage with life. Conscious disconnection and cord cutting, when practiced regularly, lead to less frequent anxiety triggers coming from the present and future. **Instead of being overwhelmed, you're actively engaging with life on your terms.**

Transmutation: Rewriting Reality

We've explored how to consciously connect and disconnect from the world around us, giving you the tools to step out of autopilot patterns and into awareness and choice. But what if there was a third option, one that didn't just allow you to disengage from stress, but actually shift it into something better? This is where transmutation comes in. Now, before you start imagining yourself joining the X-Men and developing superpowers, let's break it down into something tangible. Transmutation, in simple terms, is the process of changing something from one state into another. It's not about suppressing emotions or pretending something doesn't bother you. Instead, it's about recognizing what you feel, neutralizing it, and then **intentionally shifting** your response in a way that benefits you. This isn't just wishful thinking; it's a deliberate practice of taking back control from the external world and deciding *how* you want to feel, regardless of the circumstances.

Transmutation: The process of changing something from one state to another.

Let's go back to the example of getting stuck in traffic. Initially, I presented two different responses you could have. One where you react negatively, get frustrated, and let the stress take over. Or two, you disconnect and neutralize, taking a deep breath and accepting that the traffic is out of your control. But there's a third choice I didn't initially present: transmuting or changing your current state into a different one. While unfortunately we don't have the ability to change our physical reality in the moment, hover our vehicle out of traffic, or teleport ourselves back home, we absolutely *can* change our emotional response to it. Instead of seeing traffic as wasted time, you use it as an opportunity. Maybe you put on your favorite podcast, or listen to a song that lifts your mood, or take the time to focus on something you want to manifest. **This changes a moment of limitation into a moment of expansion.** At first, it may be difficult to shift your state, especially when emotions like anger, sadness, or frustration are strong. But the more you practice switching your perspective, the easier it becomes to turn any situation into something that benefits you.

Let's use another example to really drive home this point, going back to my sad cold cup of stale coffee. I was able to bring awareness to my present moment and then choose to connect with the coffee. Upon connecting, I realized that it no longer held joy for me anymore. But what if I wanted to bring that joy back without changing the current circumstance? Instead of heating it back up or grabbing myself a second biscotti, I decided to reconnect with it through gratitude. By observing it and asking myself to focus on one aspect I could appreciate, I switched the energy around it. So what is there to appreciate about a cold cup of coffee? Well, the caffeine, of course! As I reconnected with it, I started to focus primarily on how grateful I was that this muddy liquid was giving me that extra boost I needed in my day. Instead of feeling sad and disappointed by it, I started feeling excited and appreciative of it.

Every time you practice transmutation, you are rewiring your brain's default auto response. Instead of anxiety being your default response to uncertainty, you train your mind to see *opportunity* instead of *obstacles*. This practice reinforces a deep truth you have forgotten along the way: You are the only one in control of your life. The more you shift your perspective, the more your subconscious mind learns to seek gratitude, empowerment, and calm instead of fear and resistance. At first, it may feel forced, like you're just saying the words without feeling them. But with time, this shift becomes second nature. Eventually, you won't have to consciously "find" gratitude; it will naturally become the way you experience life. Anxiety thrives on negative reinforcement; the more you feed it, the stronger it gets. When you constantly *react* to stress, you reinforce the belief that life is happening *to you* rather than *for you*. But by choosing to connect, disconnect, and then shift your perspective, you disrupt this cycle.

Remember that every moment in life presents you with three options: Connect to it, disconnect from it, and/or transmute it. **At its core, transmutation is about mastering your own reality.** It's a skill that transforms not only your anxiety, but your entire life. When you stop letting external events dictate your emotions, you become truly free. So the next time you feel frustration, fear, or stress creeping in, remember, you are not powerless. You always have a choice. Recognize it, neutralize it, and then decide how you want to feel. Because *that* is your true superpower.

Final Notes

This chapter held some big concepts. Let's pause for a moment and take a deep breath. Check in with yourself. How are you feeling right now? What's showing up in your body and your mind?

Through the ReNU framework, we've discovered how powerful it is to first recognize anxiety, neutralize its intensity, and then consciously utilize its energy to your advantage. This practice empowers you to then actively engage in Vibrational Navigation, choosing when and how to connect or disconnect from aspects of your reality. By doing so, you're reclaiming your power, strengthening your sense of trust, and reinforcing your self-worth. You truly are the bridge between your current reality and the one you've always wanted. **Anxiety, when understood and harnessed, becomes less of an obstacle and more of a guideline, signaling moments of opportunity and growth.** Instead of running on autopilot and reacting out of fear, you're consciously navigating your experience, deciding what serves your highest good, and gently releasing what doesn't. **At its core, anxiety comes from the discomfort of uncertainty and a desire for control.** By bringing greater awareness to your thoughts and choices, you disrupt anxiety's cycle. **By doing so, you're not just reacting anymore; you're *thoughtfully responding*.** Every conscious choice, every mindful connection or disconnection, creates a ripple effect that gradually transforms your life.

The journey of consciously assessing and reshaping your reality is a profound act of empowerment. You now hold the tools to navigate your reality, shifting not only your emotional reactions, but also your neurological patterns. A simple thought of gratitude or an intentional moment of connection can shift your entire day. Anxiety isn't just happening to you; you're now equipped to decide how you want to experience it. With these tools in hand, what new choices will you make moving forward?

Key Chapter Takeaways

- Future anxiety happens because your brain can't pinpoint the source of the problem so it makes up scenarios in an attempt to find solutions and keep you safe.
- The ReNU strategy is your greatest tool in stopping anxiety cycles in the moment and taking your power back from anxiety in the future.
- Vibrational Navigation (connection, disconnection, and transmutation) allows you to make conscious choices in how you connect with the world around you, then empowers you to change the impact of the situations in your life.

Key Action Steps

- Recognize when your mind first starts feeling anxious.
- Create a sense of calm through a focus on safety and breath.

- Observe the anxious thoughts without an emotional response.
- Set an alarm on your phone to practice connecting, disconnecting, and transmuting physical and emotional aspects of your day.

Client Case Study
Caroline the Overthinker

Caroline's mind was a 24/7 disaster simulation. If there was even the smallest thing to worry about, her brain had already written, directed, and produced an entire worst-case scenario movie about it. What if she lost her job? What if something terrible happened to her family? What if she made a mistake that she didn't even realize she made, and it ruined her life?! And so the loop continued, day and night. Caroline was exhausted, she wasn't sleeping, she wasn't present, and she felt trapped.

When we started working together, I told her something she wasn't expecting: "Your anxiety is actually trying to help you."

She gave me a look, and said, "What!? No, it's ruining my life and needs to stop."

"Your mind isn't broken; it's just trying to problem-solve without a clear problem *to* solve. Your mind does this to make you feel safe and in control. It's not a bad thing." Once she heard this, it opened something up in her, a new perspective of sorts. I began teaching her how to simply observe the spiraling thoughts, rather than reacting to them. One week, she came back with a look of accomplishment on her face. She said, "Well, I tried that thing that you said and observed my thoughts and the emotions that came with it."

"And . . . ?" I prompted.

"And, weirdly enough, it worked—at first, anyway. I caught myself starting to spiral and felt strong enough to walk beside the thought into the worst-case scenario. It was intense, as you mentioned it would be, but after a while, the emotion decreased and that particular fear hasn't come up since." Once she nailed down recognition and neutrality, we moved on to Vibrational Navigation.

"Throughout every moment of your day, whether in your mind or outside of your body, you are given a choice—to connect, disconnect, or transmute," I said. "Here are three questions to ask yourself in moments of overwhelm and uncertainty:

"Am I going to connect with this thought and let it shape me?

"Am I going to disconnect from it because it doesn't serve me?

"Or am I going to transmute it and shift it into something higher?"

The change wasn't immediate, but steadily, her mental storm started to calm, the nighttime spirals lost their grip, and she stopped believing every thought her anxiety threw at her. I saw her become more empowered, more grounded, and overall more free right in front of my eyes.

If you've ever felt stuck in a loop of anxious overthinking, **remember that not every thought is a fact.**

You don't have to react to everything your mind throws at you. Your conscious awareness is what holds the key to your true freedom. So ask yourself, "What am I connecting to in this moment, and how is that making me feel?"

Chapter 6

The Anxiety Detox: From Fear to Trust

Hey Anxiety Ally,

Have you ever experienced a moment where you just let go, truly let go, and trusted? Usually, these moments don't come easily. They show up when you're at your breaking point, in a place of pure desperation. It happens when you're so drained, so overwhelmed, that you simply can't muster the energy to worry anymore. You're forced to surrender, and in that moment, something shifts.

It's freeing, isn't it? There's a sense of peace that washes over you, like you've been carrying a heavy load and finally set it down. It makes you wonder, what if I could feel this free all the time? For a brief moment, you get a glimpse of what life could feel like without anxiety constantly pulling at you.

But then, as if on cue, the anxiety creeps back in. The fear, the worry, the overthinking, it grabs hold and drags you back into the cycle. It's frustrating, because you've felt what it's like to trust and let go. You've seen the possibility, yet it feels just out of reach.

Trust and surrender are powerful, sustainable solutions for overcoming anxiety at its core. But let's be real—applying this in everyday life isn't as simple as flipping a switch. It takes awareness, practice, and a whole lot of patience. Trust doesn't happen overnight, especially when your mind is conditioned to focus on control, worst-case scenarios, and the constant need to "fix" things.

In this chapter, we're going to dive into what it really means to let go and trust. Not just in those moments of desperation, but as a practice you can integrate into your daily life. We'll explore how surrendering isn't about giving up or being passive; it's about choosing to release the grip of fear and stepping into a state of flow. It's about finding freedom in the present moment, even when the future feels uncertain.

If you're tired of being tossed around by fear and worry, this chapter is your invitation to something different, a life where trust becomes your anchor, and letting go becomes your superpower. It's not always easy, but it's worth it. And I'll walk you through every step of the process.

Let's get started. Freedom is closer than you think.

Trust

We've spent this entire book breaking down the mechanics of anxiety, where it comes from, why it happens, and how to navigate it through *awareness*, *neutrality*, *connection*, and *transmutation*. But now, we arrive at one of the last, and perhaps most important, steps: *trust*.

At its core, anxiety thrives in the absence of trust. When we don't trust ourselves, we second-guess every decision. When we don't trust others, we micromanage and overanalyze interactions. And when we don't trust life, we try to control every outcome, convinced that uncertainty equals danger. Realistically, most of us believe that we are trusting people. But trust isn't just about having faith in others; it's about how much faith we have in **ourselves, our instincts, and the flow of life itself.** If anxiety has a grip on you, chances are, your relationship with trust has some cracks in it.

Let's go ahead and kick off this chapter with a quiz. You may think you're a trusting person, but sometimes these mechanisms are so deeply embedded you don't even realize when you're stuck. Ready to find out?

Quiz: How Much Do You Trust?

Instructions: Answer each question. At the end, tally up how many a's, b's, and c's you picked.

1. **When faced with uncertainty, how do you typically respond?**
   a. I try to control every detail to ensure a specific outcome.
   b. I feel uneasy but remind myself that things will unfold as they should.
   c. I trust that everything is happening for a reason, even if I don't understand it.

2. **How often do you take time to reflect on your higher purpose?**
    a. Rarely: I focus more on the tangible, day-to-day tasks.
    b. Occasionally: When I feel overwhelmed or stuck, I'll tune in.
    c. Regularly: I often remind myself that my soul chose this journey for a reason.
3. **When things don't go as planned, how do you feel?**
    a. Frustrated and anxious: I feel like I failed or could have done something better.
    b. Disappointed but open to the idea that there may be a reason behind the setback.
    c. Peaceful: I trust that this is guiding me toward a better outcome.
4. **How often do you seek external validation or reassurance in decision-making?**
    a. Very often: I struggle to make decisions without others' input.
    b. Sometimes: I check in with others, but I trust my gut most of the time.
    c. Rarely: I trust myself to make aligned decisions without needing external approval.

5. **When you think about surrendering control, what comes up for you?**
   a. Fear: I worry that things will fall apart if I'm not in control.
   b. Resistance: I know it's important, but it's challenging to let go.
   c. Relief: Surrendering feels like a natural and freeing choice.

Your Score & Results

Mostly A's: Learn to Let Go

You may lean toward control as a coping mechanism for anxiety. This can make it difficult to trust yourself fully. Reflect on how letting go of control could create space for peace and alignment.

Mostly B's: Work in Progress

You're working on balancing trust and control. You may still feel moments of resistance but are open to the idea of surrender and trusting in the bigger picture.

Mostly C's: Well on Your Way

You embody trust in the flow of life and yourself. You understand that life's unfolding is divinely orchestrated, allowing you to experience greater inner peace.

Just trust the universe, they say; it'll work out, they say . . . but then it doesn't work out, and in fact, sometimes life gets worse after trusting. You might think, *No thanks. I'll go back to micromanaging, overthinking, and planning. At least that way I know for sure everything will be anticipated, which will minimize the unexpected, which then decreases the possibility of disappointment and emotional turmoil.*

What's really funny about anxiety is that, at a certain point, **our desire to avoid unwanted situations ends up creating them.** While trying to define this effect, I came across research from a psychologist named Daniel Wegner. He coined it the "ironic process theory," or the "white bear effect."

The White Bear Effect

You are told to *not* think about a white bear. You try very hard to push that thought away. Despite your greatest efforts, the idea of a white bear keeps popping into your head more and more frequently. The act of trying to avoid the thought ironically reinforces it, making it harder to escape.

In life, and for highly anxious people, the white bear effect is a chronic spiral. It's like the mental version of the Chinese finger trap; the more you pull, the more you are stuck, but when you relax you are able to get free. I find that when I'm stuck in an anxiety loop where I worry about the thing I don't want to have happen, I end up focusing on it more and therefore worry about it more. I get frustrated and try to push the feeling down, rather than letting go of it, and relaxing. Because of this, I envy the people who are detached.

The ones who don't see the fingerprints on the fridge, who don't feel the emotions of their kids or the chaos of society. The detached ones seem like the least anxious ones. They deal with life as it arises with no forethought or afterthought about it. Similar to having a cushy government job, you clock in at 9 AM and clock out at 5 PM and call it a day of good work, go home, and spend time with the family. These days, that separation and compartmentalization doesn't exist like it used to. Our private, public, family, and work lives seem to just meld together.

I often wonder whether the detached people are choosing to be that way or if they are naturally that way. I wonder if I could also choose to be detached. Part of me thinks they all might just be so ungrounded they aren't connected long enough to feel and know all the things we do. Maybe they do float back in every once in a while, and get hit with a wave of anxiety, and then check back out because it's easier. I don't know because I've never been that way.

If I could choose to be a certain way, **I would want to maintain my awareness but let go of the *worry* around the awareness.** I've spent many years rolling these questions and observations around in my head. And I've come to one big question that I will attempt to solve in this very chapter: **What is the best state of being we could exist in?**

Knowing Versus Not Knowing

When I first began tapping into my extrasensory abilities, it felt as if the world had opened up in a completely new way.

I could read a client's auric field, uncover hidden emotional blocks, or even connect with someone's deceased loved one to bring them closure. One of the most practical and fascinating ways I used my gifts, however, was to understand the *why* behind life's events.

Extrasensory Abilities: The ability to tap into energy or information that exists beyond the physical realm.

For example, let's say you get into a car accident. On a surface level, the explanation is simple: Maybe the driver behind you was texting and rear-ended your car. But could there be a bigger reason behind it? Perhaps it served as a wake-up call for the other driver to pay more attention. Maybe it created an opportunity for you to get a new car completely covered by insurance. When we start exploring the deeper layers of even the most mundane experiences, life becomes far more intentional. Nothing feels random, and every moment holds potential insight.

In 2013, I had an experience that reinforced this perspective. That day, I had an inexplicable feeling that I needed to go to a local market near my house. Before heading out, I put eighty dollars in my pocket, far more cash than I would typically take, but something told me I would need it. I hopped on my motorcycle and rode over, convinced that I would find something I had to buy. But after an hour of wandering through the booths, nothing called to me. Confused, I left the market and got back on my bike, heading home.

That's when I got stuck in a brutal traffic jam. The heat

was unbearable, and I felt like I was melting in my gear. Frustrated, I decided to turn around and take another route. I looked both ways and went to make my turn when, out of nowhere, a man on a bicycle collided with my motorcycle. Shocked, I dropped my bike.

Immediately, I felt like it was my fault. I hadn't seen him coming, and I felt awful. We both pulled into a nearby parking lot to talk. As I took off my helmet, apologizing profusely, I saw him clearly for the first time. From the way he was dressed, it appeared as though he was experiencing homelessness or just really struggling financially. In that moment, I knew; the cash wasn't for me. It was for him. I reached into my pocket and handed him the eighty dollars, telling him, "I now understand why I had this money on me today—it was for you." At first he hesitated, insisting he couldn't take it. But after I insisted, he finally accepted it, his eyes filled with gratitude. He told me he'd been having a *really* rough week and that I had no idea how much this meant to him.

That moment changed my understanding of trust and alignment. If I hadn't followed that internal nudge, if I hadn't carried that exact amount of money, if I hadn't turned around in traffic, we never would have crossed paths. It was a perfect example of how **trusting *without needing to know* can lead to beautiful, synchronistic moments.**

The Downside of Needing to Know

Understanding the deeper meaning behind events can be incredibly empowering. But I soon learned that *needing to know everything* could become just as detrimental as knowing nothing at all. For a time, I became obsessed with uncovering the meaning behind *all aspects of life*. If a pillow fell off the couch, I would question why. *Was this a sign that I'm unsupported in my life? Was it a message to let go because my ex bought it? Or was it something even deeper?* It reached the point where my friends were frustrated with me. If they tripped over their own feet or failed a test, I wouldn't express sympathy. Instead, I'd immediately ask, "What lesson are you learning?"

The breaking point came during a weekend getaway with a friend. We had rented a cozy, remote cabin, the perfect escape from life. The first morning, as I lay in bed, I looked up at the wooden ceiling bathed in sunlight. And that's when I saw them—millions of tiny dust particles floating through the air like glitter. At first, I was mesmerized. But then my mind started racing. *What are these particles? Dust? Dead skin cells from the previous tenants? Tiny mites? Am I breathing this in? Are they inside me now?*

I spiraled into a full-blown panic attack. I quickly left the cabin to catch my breath and went on a long hike through the woods. When I returned, the dust was gone, nowhere to be seen, and I felt instant relief. But a few days later I realized that the dust never actually disappeared. It was still there. I just couldn't see it without the sunlight hitting it.

This was a *huge* breakthrough for me. That dust had always been in the air, whether I saw it or not. The only thing that changed was my *awareness* of it. This realization applied far beyond that moment. It applied to *everything*. Awareness is key—to an extent. So what's the perfect balance? Where can we land that allows us to fully experience life *without* overwhelming ourselves?

The place where I feel most at peace, least anxious, and most fulfilled is a delicate balance between knowing and not knowing. And the one thing that allows me to navigate this space? **Trust.** How many times have you confided in someone about your anxiety, only to hear them say, "You just need to trust more"? It's easy to say, but hard to do.

That's why this chapter is dedicated to deepening your understanding of trust, not as a vague concept, but as a practical, embodied state of being. When you learn how to truly trust, you no longer need to control everything, you no longer feel consumed by uncertainty, and most importantly, **you realize that you are always supported, even when you don't have all the answers.**

Free Will Versus Destiny

One of the biggest questions I asked myself at a young age was, "How does the universe work?" I wanted the keys to understanding my own existence, my purpose, and the meaning behind life itself. Through years of deep meditation and altered states of consciousness, I kept receiving the same answer: "You create this reality."

At first, this response felt overwhelming. How could I be creating everything? What about fate, divine intervention, or the things that seemed completely out of my control? The idea that I was the creator of my own experience felt both empowering and intimidating. It took me years to unpack it, to truly understand how reality is shaped by both our choices (free will) and life's bigger plan (destiny).

The reason this is important, especially when it comes to anxiety, is because it directly ties into our ability to trust. When we learn to trust, not just ourselves, but the balance between free will and destiny, we unlock a level of freedom that anxiety can never touch. We begin to see that life isn't just something happening *to* us, but something happening *through* us. In the sections ahead, I'll break down the difference between free will and destiny, how both exist simultaneously, and how embracing this balance allows us to step out of fear and into deep, unwavering trust.

Free Will

Free will is our greatest asset as humans. It's the ability to make choices entirely on our own. While there may be societal expectations, laws, or personal limitations we impose on ourselves, the fundamental truth remains: **We always have the power to choose.**

Free Will: The divine ability to make choices independent of external control, karmic contracts, or programmed belief systems.

This realization should be liberating, yet we usually feel stuck, weighed down by the responsibilities and structures of the world around us. The noise of everyday life drowns out the fact that, in any given moment, we hold the steering wheel of our own reality.

Think back to childhood, when life's possibility felt limitless. We were told we could be anything we wanted, a firefighter, an astronaut, even the president. As kids, we made choices based purely on what excited us the most. Somewhere along the way, however, that innate sense of freedom started to disappear. Fast-forward twenty-five years later, and many of us wake up in careers we never dreamed of, feeling unfulfilled but unsure how we got here. How did we go from a six-year-old full of wonder to a thirty-year-old who feels stuck in a system that seems to dictate our every move?

The answer lies in choice. We still have the power we did as children, but we've been conditioned to forget it. Society encourages conformity, practicality, and playing it safe. We get so caught up in expectations that we end up choosing what feels familiar over what truly excites us. We trade in passion for predictability, often without even realizing it.

The moment you remember that your free will is always active, you reclaim your power. When you realize that you are in control of your choices, you shift from being a passenger in life to the one driving. That realization can be empowering . . . or overwhelming. Stepping back into infinite possibility can feel like ordering from a ten-page menu at a restaurant, with so many options that the sheer overwhelm pushes you to choose something safe rather than risk picking something new. The same thing happens in life. When faced with too many choices, fear and uncertainty can paralyze us, leading us to default to what's comfortable, even when comfort isn't fulfilling.

Everything in life comes down to choice. Every situation, every opportunity, every challenge is the result of a choice we either actively made or passively accepted. Taking responsibility for our choices, both good and bad, is the first step toward creating a life of freedom and fulfillment. However, free will is only one side of the equation. To fully understand how our lives unfold, we must also talk about the other force at play: destiny.

Destiny

I like to refer to destiny as contracts or blueprints. Before moving ahead, let me define some terms so we're all on the same page.

The word *destiny* often implies a God-given higher path, but that's not quite how it works. We all have predestined contracts, which are specific life experiences our souls have chosen to fulfill in order to learn particular lessons. The entire purpose of incarnation itself is to experience limitation and evolve through it. Many of our life contracts are rooted in our soul's need for experience. For example, if you need to learn the lesson of financial lack, you might lose a significant amount of money in this incarnation. Maybe it happens through theft, a bad night of gambling, a divorce, or a risky investment. No matter how it unfolds, it was written into your contract to teach you what financial loss feels like so that you can learn from it. So many people assume that our contracts are written by a higher being or source, but it's actually you, and your own soul, who decides your life blueprint before incarnating. Before each lifetime, you meet with your spirit guides to determine what lessons you need to experience next, then choose how they will play out.

Soul: An eternal, energetic being of consciousness that exists beyond the physical body, experiencing many lifetimes to evolve, learn, and expand its awareness.

Spirit Guides: Nonphysical beings, often souls who are highly evolved, ancestors, angels, or members of your spirit family, who assist, guide, protect, and support you throughout your life journey, helping you navigate challenges and align with your blueprints/contracts.

Destiny/Contracts/Blueprints: A pre-agreed-upon set of experiences decided by your soul and spirit guides before coming to Earth.

Incarnation: The process by which a soul chooses to enter a physical body in order to explore set experiences in order to learn and grow.

Timeline: A potential path or trajectory of reality based on energy, choices, and frequency. Timelines are not fixed; they shift and change depending on individual and collective consciousness.

When I first started exploring this concept, I felt trapped by the idea that every aspect of my life was predestined. I would try to rebel against my own life contracts by making random, unexpected choices just to prove that I was the one in control. At the time, I assumed someone else had made these predestined choices for me. Looking back, I see how misguided that was. Now I understand that while the big experiences in our lives like relationships, children, or a new job are contracted, the smaller, day-to-day choices are governed by our free will. However, when we have moments where destiny seems to override our personal choices, it can create confusion and inner conflict.

So, what does any of this have to do with anxiety? When we believe that everything in our life depends solely on our decisions, the pressure can feel overwhelming. On the other hand, if we believe that a higher power dictates our entire life, we feel powerless. The key is to integrate both free will and destiny into our lives. This helps us to understand that the big things are destined to happen, and that even when life moments are challenging, they are always aligned to our highest good and are there to help us grow. With this perspective, we can navigate life's challenges with greater ease. Take parenting, for example. If you're anxious about your child getting hurt while riding their bike, you might try to control the situation, limiting their time on the bike, overprotecting them with knee and elbow pads, or restricting them from riding with friends. But this anxiety doesn't just affect you; it can instill fear in your child, making them hesitant or overly cautious. Or, in defiance, they may push back and ride recklessly just to assert their own independence. This is the white bear effect in action. The more you fixate on preventing something, the more it manifests in different ways.

This is a good example of a place where you could apply the ReNU method to your worst-case-scenario fears. Then remind yourself, if a serious injury were to happen, it would be part of your child's contract. No amount of worry or control can prevent what is meant to unfold, or force something that isn't meant to happen. The same applies to your own life. Whether it's a career shift, a move, or a health challenge, you can set intentions, but your soul contracts will ultimately guide you. **Sometimes, life isn't about micromanaging to mitigate risk; it's about surrendering and trusting that you are being guided beyond what you are able to witness.**

So, what does all of this actually mean for your life and your anxiety? It means that even though some aspects of your journey may have been set in motion before you got here, you still have full control over how you navigate them.

Think of it like this: **Destiny is the road, but free will is how you drive.** Some roads may have sharp turns, uphill climbs, or unexpected detours—these are the soul lessons you agreed to experience. But you get to decide how you show up for them. Do you speed through in a panic, fearing every bump? Or do you slow down, trust the path, and learn to enjoy the ride?

Anxiety thrives when we believe that we are powerless passengers, being thrown into situations beyond our control. When you recognize that you have the power to shift, grow, and choose your response, life becomes less about the fear of the unknown and more about curiosity for what's ahead. This perspective shift is everything. It's how you move from anxiety into empowerment, from feeling like life is something happening to you, to realizing you are an active creator in every moment. The future is not set in stone. It's a fluid, evolving experience, shaped by your choices, your energy, and your willingness to step into your power. The more you trust that you are meant to be exactly where you are, with full freedom to shape what comes next, the less anxiety will control your experience. **At the end of the day, you're both the writer and the main character of your life's story.** Some plot points may already be written, but how the story unfolds? That's entirely up to you.

Everything Happens for a Reason

We can only ever accept and let go after we have overcome our emotional reaction around the thoughts in our mind. **As sugar is food to parasites, fear is food to anxiety.** Through consciously observing the uncomfortable thoughts in our mind and sensations in our body, we are able to move forward, out of the loop. You choose to stop overanalyzing and just show up with no expectation, attachments, fears, or worries. You trust that everything happens for a reason, and no matter if it's good or bad, it has something to teach us. **Instead of attempting to anticipate the blows of life and making life unbearable by sitting in that anticipation, we just show up and deal with what comes as it comes.** Instead of actively trying not to focus on the white bear, we detach from the outcome and in so doing let it walk away.

When we allow life to happen and ask ourselves questions to better understand the reason for those happenings, we maintain a state of trust. That level of trust is hard to come by, but once we have it, we finally feel free in our own minds. Life isn't always meant to be good. Life isn't supposed to be butterflies and rainbows. Life is messy and constantly changing. The more we try to attach ourselves to an expected outcome, the more challenges around that outcome we experience. As we heal the past traumas and allow ourselves to be okay with sitting in those emotions, we release the fears we have over the future. By showing up in every moment without attachment or worries around what might happen next, we ground ourselves into the precious present moment. Trust is about accepting all potential possibilities, good and bad, and knowing that we have the skills to navigate anything that comes up.

Control Versus Surrender

Anxiety, at its core, is about control—specifically, the fear of *losing* control. When we're anxious, we're desperately trying to manage outcomes, predict the future, and protect ourselves from the unknown. We tell ourselves, *If I can just figure everything out, I'll feel safe.* But the truth is, we're never going to figure it all out. Life is inherently unpredictable. And in our attempts to micromanage the chaos, we only end up creating more anxiety for ourselves. The more we resist the flow of life, the more we end up manifesting the very things we're trying to avoid. It's the classic example of the white bear effect. The harder we try to push away an unwanted thought or scenario, the more it dominates our mind.

The lesson here is simple yet profound: Control is an

illusion. **We can't control the external world, but we can control our response to it.** And that's where surrender comes in. When we let go of our need to control every outcome, we free ourselves from the roller-coaster ride of expectation and disappointment. As we create space for the universe to move through us, we allow life to unfold as it's meant to.

At the heart of surrender is trust. Trust that the universe has your back, that everything is happening for a reason, and that even when things don't go according to plan, it's all part of a greater purpose. But trusting is hard, especially for those of us who have been let down before. It's hard to trust when you've experienced trauma, when you've faced disappointment, and when you've been hurt by life's unpredictability. That being said, trust isn't about blind faith. It's not about pretending that everything is perfect or that bad things won't happen. **Trust is about recognizing that life is a series of cycles, highs and lows, ebbs and flows, and that each experience, whether good or bad, is a necessary part of our growth.**

We talked earlier about the balance between free will and destiny. In every moment, we have the power to create our reality through our choices and intentions. But at the same time, there are certain things, big, life-altering things, that are part of our soul's blueprint. These are the moments that are predestined to shape us, to teach us, and to help us evolve. When we trust the flow of life, we stop fighting against our destiny. We stop trying to control outcomes and instead focus on showing up fully in each moment. We recognize that every experience, even the difficult ones, is part of the greater tapestry of our life. And with that trust comes a sense of peace, an acceptance that everything is happening for a reason. **When**

we let go of the need to have everything figured out, we open ourselves up to the magic of the unknown.

Radical Responsibility: The Key to Trust

If we want to fully release anxiety and embrace trust, we need to talk about responsibility. When something unexpected happens, our control systems go into overdrive, scrambling to fix, manage, or prevent what feels like chaos. The biggest issue I've seen in my own clients is that they automatically assume they are not in control in the first place, which feeds their anxiety even more. Anxiety isn't just about the unknown; **it's about believing that the unknown is dangerous.** That life is happening to us instead of through us. This is why taking responsibility for our reality is so powerful. It's not about blame or forcing control; it's about recognizing that everything in our experience, even the challenges, is part of a bigger picture.

It's easy to blame external circumstances, the person who cut you off in traffic, the job rejection, or the friend who ghosted you. But what if, instead of feeling like a victim in these moments, you saw them as reflections of something deeper? As opportunities for awareness, growth, and realignment?

Let's say someone bumps into you on the street because they're too busy texting. Your immediate reaction might be frustration. *People are so careless!* But instead of just reacting, what if you paused and asked, *Why did I bring this moment into my experience? What is it mirroring back to me?* Maybe it's a reflection of your own distraction in life, a reminder to be more present, or an opportunity to practice patience. Maybe it's showing you where you still give away your power to external situations.

When we start to see life through this lens, everything changes. Suddenly, the universe isn't against you; it's working with you. Every challenge, every setback, every frustrating moment becomes an invitation to step into a higher level of awareness. This is why trust and responsibility go hand in hand. If you're still holding on to the belief that life is random, unfair, or completely out of your control, letting go will always feel terrifying. **But when you start to take ownership of your experience, you realize that surrender isn't about losing control; it's about finally accepting that you were in control all along.** Not in a forceful, "I must manipulate everything" kind of way, but in the sense of knowing that your thoughts, emotions, and energetic state shape what you attract and how you respond.

When you take responsibility, you shift from feeling like a passenger in life to an active participant, and that's when trust becomes second nature. You're no longer afraid of what's coming next. You already know you have the power to meet it, transform it, and grow from it.

Final Notes

Anxiety has a way of convincing us that control is our only safety net. We micromanage, overanalyze, and anticipate every possible outcome in the hope of minimizing disappointment and chaos. But as we've explored, this endless cycle of resistance only reinforces the very fears we are trying to avoid. **The more we fight against uncertainty, the more trapped we become.** Like the Chinese finger trap or the white bear effect, our attempts to control life often keep us stuck in the exact situations we fear. So what if we approached life differently? What if, instead of resisting, we softened into the unknown? What if we could hold awareness without the weight of worry?

Through this chapter, we've unraveled the intricate balance between knowing and not knowing, control and surrender, free will and destiny. We've seen that trust is not about blind faith, but about understanding the flow of life, recognizing that every challenge carries a deeper purpose. **Trust is not about believing that nothing bad will happen, but knowing that whatever does happen, you are capable of navigating it.** True freedom comes when we learn to release our attachment to specific outcomes. Instead of spending extra energy bracing for impact, we can redirect it toward presence, curiosity, and alignment. We can shift from fearing uncertainty to embracing it as the very space where magic happens.

This doesn't mean we stop planning, caring, or striving for the best. It means we release the exhausting need to force life to conform to our expectations. It means we trust that even when things don't go the way we envisioned, there is a reason embedded within.

Look at your own life. How many times did things not go according to plan, only to reveal a path that was ultimately better for you? How many times have you thought something was a disaster, only to later realize it was a necessary redirection? The universe has a way of guiding us, whether we know it or not. Every choice, every delay, every obstacle is a nudge, a reminder that we are not here to control everything, but to co-create with the destiny we already chose before arriving on this planet. Trust doesn't mean you won't feel fear; it means you won't let fear dictate your every move. So the question remains: **Will you continue to grip on to the illusion of control, or will you lean into trust? Will you let the white bear walk away, or will you keep chasing it in circles?** The choice is yours, but if peace is what you seek, surrender is the doorway.

Key Chapter Takeaways

- Anxiety thrives when we lack trust. Trust in yourself, in others, and in your divine path.
- Letting go is not passive; it's an active choice to surrender control and trust your ability to handle the unknown.
- Your past challenges were lessons preparing you for your next level of growth.

Key Action Steps

- Practice Radical Responsibility: Write down a challenging experience you had in the past and get curious about how that challenge led you to new opportunities and internal growth.
- Work with the affirmation "I trust in my higher contracts. I trust that I am exactly where I need to be."
- Practice letting go of control in one small way today, whether it's delegating a task or surrendering to an outcome.

Client Case Study
Amara: From Fearful to Free

Amara had built a life around avoiding life. For years, she barely left her house. She perceived the outside world as too unpredictable, and too scary. Her brain ran a constant reel of worst-case scenarios, which led her to making the safest choice possible: making no choices at all.

When we started working together, I asked her, "When did the fear start?"

Amara looked down. "I don't know. It feels like it was always there, but after the divorce it got worse. How could I be that wrong about someone I thought I knew? It made me have doubts in all my decisions."

I explained, "Your fear isn't just about the outside world—it's about *trust*." She didn't trust people, she didn't trust herself, and she definitely didn't trust life. But I asked her, "What if you were the one who signed up for this life before you got here? What if your biggest struggles, like your divorce, were actually your soul's choice, not for punishment, but for growth?"

At first, she resisted, hard. "Why would I ever choose this?"

My response was gentle but clear. "Because your soul knows what you are capable of. It wouldn't have given you anything more than you could handle and then learn from." As we worked through it, she started putting the pieces together. Every painful experience in her life had led her somewhere important: The heartbreak taught her self-love, the betrayal taught her boundaries, and the failures led her to unexpected, better paths. The question challenged everything she had believed, and her entire mindset cracked wide open.

Amara began to understand that she wasn't being punished; she was being guided, and for the first time in decades, she felt safe again. Slowly but surely, she started venturing outside again, first just to the end of her driveway, and then the mailbox. One day she called me, beyond excited. "You won't believe it but I went to the park. I sat on a bench and I watched people walk by. I didn't even think about running home."

I smiled to myself and asked, "And how did that feel?"

There was a pause on the other end. "Scary . . . but also kind of beautiful. I watched this little girl chase a butterfly and thought, *I want to feel that free again.*" And eventually, she was. Every step, every small moment of courage, chipped away at the mental prison she had lived in for years. It was trust she was missing and trust she finally leaned into.

If you've ever felt stuck, paralyzed, or afraid to step forward, remember this: **Your life isn't happening to you; it's happening for you.** And you are stronger than your fear.

Chapter 7

Anxiety Is Your Superpower

Hey Anxiety Ally,

I see you. I know what it's like to feel like anxiety is a relentless, unpredictable force in your life. But what if I told you that anxiety isn't here to break you; it's here to wake you? What if, instead of seeing it as an enemy, you started recognizing it as your greatest superpower? Anxiety isn't just a random inconvenience; it's a heightened state of awareness, a signal, a built-in guidance system that most people just ignore. It sharpens your instincts, pushes you toward growth, and reveals where your energy is misaligned. The key isn't to silence it; it's to listen, decode, and redirect it. When you learn how to harness anxiety rather than fear it, you unlock a level of power, intuition, and clarity that most people spend their entire lives searching for. You are not broken. You are not weak. You are gifted. And it's time to reclaim that gift.

Stop and Listen

I know what you might be thinking. *Elizabeth, anxiety feels terrible! How could it possibly be a superpower?* Trust me, I've been there, heart racing, stomach churning, thoughts spiraling, wondering if I'm losing it, but what if I told you that beneath the overwhelm is your soul's direct line of communication, your own built-in spidey sense screaming out for your attention?

In this last chapter, I want to take you by the hand and show you exactly how to tune in to your anxiety, listen deeply, and turn it into the single most empowering tool you have in your emotional tool kit. Anxiety is an unseen experience and yet it is felt deeply throughout every part of our system, body, and mind. We now understand that anxiety is simply an alert system, one we rarely stop to recognize. Instead, we ignore it until the alarms ring so loud that we're left with no choice but to listen, often out of sheer desperation.

So how do we shift anxiety from an overwhelming alarm into a powerful tool that helps us navigate life? The answer lies in two simple words: *stop* and *listen*. As mentioned in previous chapters, **the negative effects of anxiety stem not from the alert itself but from our reaction to it.** What if we took a moment between the alarm and the symptoms to just stop and listen? By interrupting the cycle in its tracks and responding differently, we disrupt our automatic neurological patterns. Our brains are designed for survival. They respond with the same reactions to external triggers. This built-in predictability is there to keep us safe, but it also keeps us stuck. Any difference from our usual response feels uncertain, and scary. Typically, we react to anxiety in one of two ways: We either distract and dissociate, or we hyper-focus on the symptoms, making them worse. To break free from this subconscious loop, we must observe with our conscious mind. Just by observing it, we reclaim our power. **This simple act of *presence* gives us the ability to choose how we respond.** That choice is the difference between an automatic freak-out and the awareness of an intuitive alert.

If anxiety is simply awareness misunderstood, then stopping and listening is the only way to truly understand it. The true shift with anxiety is learning how to harness it for good. Learning how to listen to its messages rather than assume they are something to fear.

When anxiety symptoms emerge, take a moment to *question the anxiety itself.* Instead of getting lost in it, ask, "Where are you coming from?" Try to pinpoint whether it's linked to the past, present, or future. For instance, if you suddenly feel anxious, but nothing obvious is happening in the present moment, reflect on whether it's connected to something unresolved from the past. By identifying the source, you can then take steps to resolve it using the ReNU strategy. Recognize that the anxiety is present. Neutralize it instead of reacting; lean in to the stored emotions. Allow yourself to feel them fully, without resistance. And then, utilize that moment of awareness by shifting your perspective. Ask yourself what you are learning from that challenging moment. Reflect and gain access to new insights around your own life lessons. **Don't wait for life to teach you; show up ready to learn from life.** This allows us to expedite the challenges we go through—no longer will you be hit with the same obstacles over and over again. If you can show up presently for all life has to offer, your anxiety doesn't have to keep sounding the same alarm, hoping that one day you will pay attention and learn.

The Power of Past Anxiety—Your Teacher

In many ways, past anxiety is like an internal teacher telling you about yourself—or a therapist constantly nudging you to release old burdens. As we covered in chapter 3, anxiety rooted in the past stems from ignored or suppressed alarms, whether we meant to ignore them or not. Unresolved traumas and emotions remain in our energy field, waiting for us to acknowledge them. These traumas need the same thing anxiety does: *our attention*. Our bodies create physical pain to force us to focus, and our minds generate unnecessary fears to call in our awareness. Every symptom we experience is simply a call for conscious attention.

When we provide ourselves with a safe space to process these unresolved energies, the tension eases, and the alarms finally turn off. But how do we know when we've fully healed the past? The answer isn't always clear. In my experience, there are two key indicators:

1. In moments of quiet, like when you're showering or lying in bed, does your mind wander back to old experiences or unresolved situations?

2. When you think about the most challenging moments of your life, do you still feel an emotional or physical reaction?

If you answered yes to both, there's still healing work to be done. If you answered no to both, it's a good sign you've cleared a lot of old energy and are ready to move forward. (And, as mentioned in chapter 5, experiencing more future anxiety can also be an indication that the traumas of the past are healed.) However, healing isn't a one-and-done event. Life constantly presents new challenges, which require more healing and awareness. The key is not to accumulate unresolved emotions over time but to integrate healing as an ongoing practice.

For example, if you and your partner have an argument but never take the time to process and resolve it, that emotional energy lingers. The next day, it becomes part of your past, a tiny trauma now stored in your system. It might not seem significant at first, especially if you distract yourself from it. But eventually, those unresolved emotions will resurface as anxiety symptoms. It could happen the next day, or it might accumulate over time and hit you unexpectedly months later. Either way, it remains within you until it's fully addressed. And no, just because a trauma involves another person doesn't mean you need them in order to resolve it. Your healing is your responsibility. This is where the concept of radical responsibility comes in. If you neglect these accumulated energies, you become like the oversaturated sponge, unable to absorb anything new without overflowing. The smallest unexpected event can send you into emotional overload because you're already carrying the weight of so much unresolved energy from the past.

Think of past anxiety as a helpful messenger reminding you to take an energetic shower, letting go of what no longer serves you. Rather than waiting years to clear stored emotions and traumas, make it a habit to process them regularly, especially after a particularly stressful week or month. Releasing these energies is as simple as bringing your conscious awareness to them. It's like tidying up your home every day instead of letting the mess build until it becomes overwhelming. If we can learn to stop and listen to these signals in the moment, we'll never have to backtrack again. By allowing past anxiety and that spidey sense alarm to bring our awareness into what needs to be healed, it starts to work for us, rather than against us. It helps us to heal deep-seated energies we may not have been aware of before and learn lessons we no longer need to repeat. In this way, past anxiety becomes our teacher—an ally, not an enemy.

The Power of Present Anxiety—Your Compass

Imagine for a moment that you are completely telepathic. Every person you interact with—your in-laws, your boss, even complete strangers—you can read their thoughts and feel their emotions. No longer are you left trying to read between the lines. Instead, you see straight through the conversation into something far deeper and far more complex. What would you do with this ability? How could you practically integrate it into your life so that it works for you?

Present anxiety functions in exactly this way. It's the hidden messaging system behind our physical interactions. By showing up and listening to the very first spidey sense alert, we can gather valuable information that can **help us navigate reality with more clarity; present anxiety becomes like an energetic compass.** As we explored in chapter 2, the energy of the planet is shifting, making us all more sensitive to unseen forces, which only adds to the overstimulation of our environments. The alert itself is trying to bring our awareness to the unseen so that we can be informed. The issue arises when we ignore our spidey sense, leading to overwhelm and confusion about why we feel so overstimulated.

Picture this: During your workday, you suddenly feel a twisting sensation in your gut. Instead of brushing it off, you pause and ask yourself, "Where is this feeling coming from?" You realize something shifted during your meeting with your boss. She seemed distracted while you discussed the upcoming merger. Now that you've pinpointed the moment your anxiety was triggered, you can follow up with the question, "Is this alert signaling something positive or negative?" Take a moment to tune in to your body's response. You may feel a flutter in your solar plexus. Does it feel like excitement or nervous tension? Simply be aware of the sensation without judgment. Next, ask yourself, "Does this alert have to do with me, or someone around me?" Once again, pause and feel into the response. If your attention naturally drifts back to your boss, then it's likely that you are picking up on *her* emotions rather than your own. This would be a good time to visualize yourself cutting the energetic cords between you. Upon doing so, you should feel immediate relief. If you don't, there may be something deeper within you that still needs attention.

Again, anxiety is just your spidey sense trying to inform you. However, not all information is valid or useful to you. This is why it's essential to develop the ability to listen to what your anxiety is telling you and then determine:

1. Is this information something I need to hold on to?
2. Is this message meant for me?
3. How do I want to respond to this alert?

Deciphering your spidey sense alerts takes time, patience, and a heightened level of awareness. However, like any skill, the more you practice, the easier it becomes. Eventually, this awareness will be automatic, and you won't need to stop and question every alert because the information will just be available to you. By doing this over and over again, you are actively reprogramming your mind to stop reacting to the spidey sense alarm as something negative and instead recognize it as valuable insight. When it comes to present-moment anxiety, much of the information we receive isn't even about us. Instead, it's often residual energy from those around us. While not every alert holds crucial or actionable information, it is a powerful reminder of your ability to feel and connect beyond the physical world.

The skill of sensing beyond the physical can be applied to all sorts of life interactions. When a friend sends a quick, dismissive text, ask yourself, *What are they really feeling? Is there something I can say that would support them?* Instead of taking their response at face value, take a moment to tune in to the energy behind their words. The same approach applies in customer service where you interact with people daily. Practice your ability to engage in Vibrational Navigation by consciously connecting with those around you. Doing so allows you to gain a deeper understanding of where they are emotionally and what they may need from you. This skill can help you impress your boss by anticipating needs and taking initiative before a direction is given. You can also apply this awareness in team meetings by noticing who seems anxious, disengaged, or energized, and offering a simple word of encouragement to someone who may be struggling. In parenting, when your child acts out or withdraws, you can pause and feel into what's truly going on beneath their behavior; are they overwhelmed, scared, or just needing reassurance? Responding to the energy rather than the surface behavior builds deeper trust. When we can show up and feel into the energetic interactions between the physical ones, we create more alignment and flow where there wasn't any before.

Not to mention that in a world flooded with AI-generated content and deepfake videos of famous people saying triggering things, our ability to understand beyond our five senses is more important than ever. We can no longer afford to rely solely on what we see or hear; we must *feel* what is true. That being said, it's important to balance connection with disconnection. Pay attention to your daily inputs and outputs. It's empowering to show up and know things without being told, but it's equally important not to carry that knowledge with you after the interaction is over.

When understood and harnessed, anxiety can help you navigate life more effectively than any guidebook ever could.

The Power of Future Anxiety—Your Creative Tool

Future anxiety is pretty wild. Our spidey sense goes off, triggering our brain to search frantically for a problem to fix. But when it can't find one, it creates one. Suddenly we are consumed with vivid worst-case scenarios. We know logically that they aren't real, and yet they feel so real that our bodies respond as if they are actually happening. The human mind, as intelligent and complex as it is, still operates on a very basic survival mechanism: to solve the problem, eliminate the threat, and ensure survival. But what happens if there is no actual problem in the moment? What if the threat is nothing more than your mind creating scarcity? Future anxiety loops are so powerful that they can trigger a full-on cognitive and biological response, for absolutely no reason. There is no immediate danger or crisis unfolding in the present moment. and yet we feel the anxiety as if we are standing face-to-face with an impending disaster. So how do we break free from these mental loops and transform them into one of our greatest superpowers?

The first step is to neutralize the emotional charge that these mental images create. As I've talked about before, the key is through acceptance. If there is a particular future scenario that triggers you the most, take the time to observe it objectively. Replay it in your mind until the emotional intensity fades. The more you do this, the less power it holds over you. Next, we deepen our trust in the flow of life by remembering a fundamental truth: Our biggest challenges are contracted experiences, written into our soul's blueprint long before we chose this incarnation. They cannot be avoided or changed; they are our destiny. No amount of mental preparation, no level of "expecting the worst," will shield us from life's toughest moments. The struggles that shape us the most always arrive unannounced. There is no planning ahead or preemptive suffering that will lessen their impact. **Your greatest struggles are your destiny, and they are also your greatest teachers.** If life were always good, if everything were easy, we would never grow or evolve. By accepting this as a reality, by truly surrendering to the idea that we are exactly where we need to be, we reclaim our power. We remind ourselves that while we may not control what happens, we do control how we respond. Through that realization, we find our strength.

Once we anchor this truth deep within us, something shifts. We develop an inner trust so profound that our mind no longer feels the need to micromanage the unknown. Anxiety begins to diminish and the need to control dissolves. Only then, once we are free from fear, can we consciously use future anxiety as a tool for *creation*. We can acknowledge that **all possibilities exist, not just the scary ones.**

Here's the most fascinating part about future anxiety: It proves how powerful our imagination is. We can think of a worst-case scenario so vividly that our physical and energetic bodies respond as if it were truly happening. So what if we harnessed that power for something good? What if, instead of spiraling into fearful realities, we started consciously imagining possible *positive* outcomes? Once you've observed and neutralized your fearful projections, ask yourself, "What is the best that could happen?" Think about the best-case scenario for your day tomorrow, or maybe for that meeting next week. Imagine yourself winning that race, or buying that new car, or convincing your boss you should get a raise. Imagine yourself completely anxiety free, able to go about the world with full trust and awareness. Let yourself fully embody these scenarios. Feel the excitement in your core and let the emotions uplift you instead of paralyze you.

Your mind is one of the most powerful tools in existence. Future anxiety, when properly understood, is simply an invitation to awareness of life's potential. It is a wake-up call, not to obsess over what could go wrong, but to consciously choose where you want your energy to flow. **Your life flows where your focus goes.** Future anxiety is really pointing you toward a space of infinite creation. If you show up, if you redirect your focus from the bad possibilities to the good, if you intentionally shift your thoughts, what could you manifest? At the end of the day, anxiety is not your enemy; it's your invitation to manifest something greater.

Final Notes

When we first began this journey, anxiety felt like a force outside of our control. It was happening to us. It overwhelmed us and dictated our thoughts, our emotions, and our choices. Anxiety has long been seen as a burden, something to fight against, suppress, or eliminate. It has been labeled as the enemy pulling us away from peace, a sign that something is wrong with us.

It should be clear now that we have been viewing it all wrong. Anxiety isn't something to fear; it's something to understand. If we don't do the work to understand the source of where it's coming from, then it will always lead our mind into confusion and spiral. So how do we go about changing our perception and reaction to this thing? We choose to show up and listen.

Through every chapter of this book, we've explored anxiety as an alert system, a spidey sense, and now, a superpower waiting to be reclaimed. Anxiety is your subconscious trying to send you information. It is your intuition lighting up, your spidey sense whispering, or sometimes shouting, "Hey! There's something you need to pay attention to." We now understand that the root cause of anxiety comes from many directions—the past, present, and future. Each direction carries a different message, and each has the potential to transform our lives.

Now we see anxiety for what it really is. **A gift. A strength. A superpower.** Anxiety was never meant to be feared or suppressed. It was meant to be understood. By learning to work *with* anxiety rather than against it, you step into a reality where you no longer feel controlled by your thoughts, but instead, choose them with intention. And that is the ultimate shift. Your past anxiety is your teacher, guiding you toward deep healing. Your present anxiety is your compass, sharpening your intuition. And your future anxiety is your creative tool, showing you the power of your own mind to manifest anything you can imagine. When you stop fearing anxiety, it stops having control over you. When you start *listening* to its messages, it becomes one of your greatest assets. And when you learn to redirect its energy, you unlock an entirely new way of moving through the world. You are no longer a victim of your mind. You are the master of it.

Key Chapter Takeaways

- Anxiety is a *guidance system*, a spidey sense alert helping you navigate life, not something to fear.
- Reprogram your reaction to anxiety; when we stop and listen, we can begin utilizing it as a tool to gain access to valuable information.
- Your mind creates your reality—if you can imagine the worst, you can also imagine and manifest the best.

Key Action Steps

- **Pause and Identify:** Ask yourself, "Is this anxiety about the past, present, or future? What is it telling me?"
- **Neutralize and Accept:** Observe anxious thoughts without fear; remind yourself that you put challenges on your path in order to learn and grow.
- **Redirect and Create:** Shift your focus from worst-case scenarios to best-case outcomes; through awareness and repetition, train your mind to expect success.

Client Case Study
Sophia: Turning Anxiety into a Superpower

Sophia was done fighting. She spent years battling anxiety, trying to shut it down, push it away, or fix it. No matter what she tried, it was always there. "I just . . . want my mind to stop," she told me in our first session. I could feel the exhaustion in her voice. It was clear that this was someone who had been at war with herself for way too long.

So I asked her, "What if anxiety isn't something to get rid of, but something to observe?"

Sophia asked, "Wait, what? What do you mean?"

"I mean . . . what if it's not the enemy? What if it's just a messenger trying to tell you something?"

No one had ever suggested that to Sophia before. "Everyone just tells me to manage it, or breathe through it, or 'stay positive,' but that never works—it always comes back."

I sighed, gathering my words. "That's because your anxiety doesn't want to be silenced; it wants to be heard. It's your early warning system, but if you don't understand it, it just feels like chaos." I continued to explain that anxiety had always been painted as the villain, the thing ruining her life, but what if it wasn't actually trying to hurt her? What if it was trying to guide her? I went on to say that anxiety isn't a malfunction; it's an alert system. It kicks in before your conscious mind catches up, like an early warning signal flashing. The problem was that no one had ever taught Sophia how to listen.

At first, this idea overwhelmed her. She had spent so long running from anxiety that the thought of sitting with it felt like inviting a monster to dinner. But slowly, she started observing it instead of reacting to it, and that's when things started making sense. Sophia began noticing patterns, like how certain people or situations triggered a specific gut feeling before anything even happened. For instance, when she was dating someone new, her spidey sense would go off around some guy making her feel anxious. On paper, they were a perfect match, so she ignored the signal. Then, sure enough, the red flags would start popping up. Her anxiety had been warning her the whole time; she just wasn't listening.

She also realized that sometimes her anxiety wasn't just alerting her of potentially bad situations; it was a push toward new opportunities. She wanted to make a big career shift but always felt butterflies around it. She realized that the nervous energy wasn't telling her "no"; it was excitement for what could be. She started realizing that the hard conversations she had been avoiding weren't something to fear. That tightness in her chest wasn't a warning to back away; it was a signal that she was ready to step into her power. The more she tuned in, the clearer it became: Anxiety wasn't the enemy; it was her intuition, her inner compass, her greatest gift. Through Vibrational Navigation, she learned how to decode her anxiety instead of being consumed by it. She let go of the fear that held her back and followed the signals that guided her forward. Over time, she took her power back and once again felt confident to make big decisions with the guidance of her spidey sense.

Sophia's transformation wasn't about getting rid of anxiety. It was about reclaiming it, and now, she's not afraid of it anymore—she's using it. **Anxiety isn't keeping her small; it's keeping her aware, safe, aligned, and connected to her truth.**

And for the first time in her life, she's not just surviving; she's thriving.

Conclusion: The Beginning of the Beginning

Hey Anxiety Ally,

As we come to the end of this book, I want you to know something. This isn't the end of your journey—it's just the beginning. The first page of a brand-new chapter in your life, where anxiety doesn't steer the ship anymore. You've spent so much time navigating the storms, feeling stuck, misunderstood, or even broken. But I hope by now you see what I see in you: strength, courage, and a spark of something so much bigger than fear. Every page you've read, every moment you've reflected, has taken you one step closer to reclaiming your freedom.

Sure, anxiety might still pop in from time to time, but you're no longer at its mercy. You've got the tools, the awareness, and most importantly, the **choice** *to rise above it. It doesn't define you; it's just a part of your story, not the main character. Now it's time to take everything you've learned here and bring it to life in a way that's uniquely you. Maybe that looks like standing up to your fears one small step at a time. Maybe it's finally* *saying yes to something that excites you or no to something that doesn't, or maybe it's just waking up tomorrow and remembering, "I am so much more than my anxiety." This is the beginning of a deeper relationship with yourself. So go ahead and take that next step, whatever it looks like for you. The world is waiting, and trust me, it's a lot brighter with you in it. You've got this, and even when it feels hard, know that I'm here cheering you on, every single step of the way.*

What Comes Next?

You're not broken. In fact, you experience anxiety because you are deeply connected. You pick up on subtle shifts, energy changes, and intuitive nudges that many others don't, and it's not a flaw. It's a skill, a superpower. **Anxiety is simply awareness misunderstood**, and now, after reading this book, you are no longer misunderstanding it. You know how to decode it, and you have the tools to navigate it. Most important, you understand that anxiety is not something to fear; it's something to listen to, learn from, and transform. So what kind of life are you going to choose now?

You can choose to see anxiety as a problem to suppress, or you can choose to see it as a guide leading you toward your highest evolution. You can continue running from it, or you can turn toward it with curiosity, trust, and a newfound sense of empowerment. Either way, the choice is yours.

I hope that this book has given you the knowledge to accept radical responsibility and step into your superpowers. If you're ready to get to work and really heal, in the following pages you'll find a twenty-one-day anxiety survival guide with daily prompts designed to help you anchor everything you've learned in order to experience lasting change. It's of course just the first step on a lifelong healing journey, but I'll be honored to be with you along the way.

As you close the book, I hope your anxiety is no longer giving *you* anxiety—and that is a beautiful thing.

The Twenty-One-Day Anxiety Survival Guide

Reset your mind, rewire your patterns, and reclaim your power

In this book I shared an entirely new perspective on anxiety, one that flipped the script, cracked open old beliefs, and gave you new and powerful tools to shift your reality. If you're here, you made it! But just reading about it isn't enough. Real transformation happens when you *apply* these concepts. Taking action on what you've learned will allow your brain to start rewiring. This is why I've created this twenty-one-day guide. It's designed to help you anchor everything you've learned in order to experience lasting change. I chose to make it twenty-one days long because that's the amount of time it takes to reprogram your neural pathways and create new, sustainable habits. **This isn't just another self-help challenge; it's a complete shift in the way you experience anxiety.** But in order for that transformation to truly take effect, you must commit. I challenge you to go all in. Show up for yourself every day, even if life gets busy or unpredictable. That said, if you miss a day (or three), no big deal. Just pick up where you left off and keep moving forward. This is about progress, not perfection.

What You'll Need

- This book (every day there are different activities so make sure you have this book and guide on you for reference)
- Two daily alarms (described on the next page)
- A notebook (it will be your new best friend—take it *everywhere*)
- An open mind (you're about to shift in ways you didn't expect)
- A commitment to yourself (because you deserve to thrive, not just survive)

The more effort you put in, the bigger the shift you'll experience. So no more excuses. You're in the driver's seat now—anxiety isn't here to hold you back; it's here to guide you toward your highest potential. You've read the book, you get the concepts, and now, it's time to integrate and embody them. Follow this guide for twenty-one days and watch anxiety transform into your greatest superpower.

How It Works: The Three Daily Actions That Will Rewire Your Mind

Every single day, you're going to engage in powerful activities and intentions to shift your mindset and reprogram your anxiety response. It'll take less than ten minutes a day, but those ten minutes are *everything*. They're the difference between staying stuck in old patterns and stepping into your most empowered self. Here's how you begin:

1. Set Two Daily Awareness Alarms

You'll be setting two alarms every day, one when you're most preoccupied and the other when you have a moment of quiet. **These are going to snap you out of autopilot and bring you into the present moment so that you can recognize and therefore shift your anxiety and its triggers.**

- Label one alarm "**Reflection Alarm.**" (My suggestion is either morning or evening, when you usually have time to yourself.)
- Label the other alarm "**Observation Alarm.**" (My suggestion is 1:11 PM or at midday, whenever you're usually busy.)

Refer to the daily guide for instructions on what to do once each alarm rings. What's cool about this strategy is that, over time, it helps us replace our internal spidey sense alarm with our own conscious awareness. The more we can show up consciously and take initiative, the less likely our systems will be to get our attention with the symptoms of anxiety.

These daily activities are quick but intentional. They'll take less than ten minutes, but during that time, stop what you're doing and drop into focus. The more presence you bring, the bigger the transformation. The more you put in, the more you get out. I'm going to push you to work with different aspects of your mind each day. If you're ready to get started, set those daily alarms now to go off twice a day for the next twenty-one days. Make sure you always have the book/guide with you, along with a notebook in order to document and anchor in your journey.

Pattern Disruptor: Rewiring Your Brain to Expect the Unexpected

Every day during this survival guide, you're going to shake things up. At any point, after one of your alarms goes off, or during a completely random moment, you'll make a different choice than what you usually do; each day has a daily Pattern Disruptor prompt. Why? Because when you break out of your usual patterns, you tell your brain, *Hey, we're not stuck in autopilot anymore, and now* I'm *in control.* This rewiring process helps you become more adaptable, present, and open to new possibilities, all of which directly improve self-worth and inner trust as well as reduce your overall anxiety. You'll start with small shifts (like ordering something new at a coffee shop or listening to music you don't normally choose) in week 1, but as you move forward, you'll push yourself into bigger, more unexpected actions. **The goal is to train your brain to *embrace* change instead of *fear* it.**

That said, you have the choice to either follow my Pattern Disruptor suggestion or do something completely different. The focus isn't on *what* you do; it's on making a new choice and reminding yourself that change is good.

WEEK 1: Observe and Recognize

Day 1: Start with Awareness

Reflection Alarm

- Set an intention by writing this out in your notebook: **"By committing to twenty-one days of awareness, I reclaim my power and shift my mindset beyond limiting thoughts and reactions."**
- Write it, read it, and feel it deeply. Take a moment to visualize yourself this time next month feeling mentally free and internally at peace.

Observation Alarm

- Stop and observe the moment.
- Narrate the present moment in your mind, as if describing it to a friend, your surroundings, the people, and any conversations happening.
- Document what you observe in your notebook.

Pattern Disruptor

- Make a new and unexpected choice today.
- **Suggestion:** Use your non-dominant hand for the next thirty minutes: eating, texting, and maybe even writing?
- Write down what you tried today, and make note of any physical or emotional reactions you experienced during or after.

Day 2: Safety First

Reflection Alarm

- Repeat this affirmation in your mind and also write it down: **"I am safe."**
- Tune in to how that feels in your mind and body; document anything that comes up.

Observation Alarm

- Stop and observe the moment.
- Ask yourself, **"Are there any aspects of this present moment that don't make me feel safe?"**
- Document what you observe in your notebook.

Pattern Disruptor

- Make a new and unexpected choice today.
- **Suggestion:** Order something you've never tried before from your favorite coffee shop.
- Write down what you tried today, and make note of any physical or emotional reactions you experienced during or after.

Day 3: Recognize Repeated Patterns

Reflection Alarm

- Reflect on a typical month and identify recurring anxiety triggers.
- Write down your reflections in your notebook.

Observation Alarm

- Stop what you're doing and observe the moment.
- Ask yourself, **"Is there anything in the present moment that would trigger my anxiety?"**
- Document what you observe in your notebook.

Pattern Disruptor

- Make a new and unexpected choice today.
- **Suggestion:** Sign up for a class, workshop, or meetup group you wouldn't normally attend.
- Write down what you tried today, and make note of any physical or emotional reactions you experienced during or after.

Day 4: Take the Oversaturated Sponge Quiz

Reflection Alarm

- Go to back to chapter 2 and take the Oversaturated Sponge Quiz.
- If you score high, follow up with observing where in your life you are taking on too much energy. Document what comes up in your notebook.

Observation Alarm

- Stop what you're doing and observe the moment.
- Ask yourself, **"What in my day is contributing to my overwhelm?"**
- Document what you observe in your notebook.

Pattern Disruptor

- Make a new and unexpected choice today.
- **Suggestion:** Intentionally say "no" to something you would typically say "yes" to, or vice versa if the opportunity arises.
- Write down what you tried, and make note of any differences you experienced during or after.

Day 5: Self Check-In

Reflection Alarm

- Spark a conversation with yourself. Say, **"Hey you, how are you feeling?"** Go back and forth with an open mind and curiosity. What new discoveries can you uncover?
- Document the conversation in your notebook.

Observation Alarm

- Pause and check in with your body. Use your five senses to notice the room's temperature, the texture of your clothing, the smells in the air, and the sounds in the moment.
- Use your notebook to document this check-in.

Pattern Disruptor

- Make a new and unexpected choice today.
- **Suggestion:** Listen to your least favorite genre of music for thirty minutes.
- Write down your initial response to the music; try to bring awareness to your response without reaction.

Day 6: Sit with a Memory That Feels Heavy

Reflection Alarm

- As long as you are in a quiet, safe space, find a painful memory to focus on.
- Play it over in your mind and bring awareness to the emotions you feel.
- Allow yourself to feel it all, and hold space for those feelings to come out.
- Write a journal entry reflecting on how it felt to just sit with a heavy memory.

Observation Alarm

- Stop what you're doing and observe the moment.
- Ask yourself, **"What is pulling the most amount of my focus at this moment?"**
- Document your findings.

Pattern Disruptor

- Make a new and unexpected choice today.
- **Suggestion:** Take a different route to get somewhere. It could be walking around your home, or driving back from work; take the road less traveled.
- Write down what you tried today and if you noticed any fears around that choice.

Day 7: Write and Burn a Cord-Cutting Letter

Reflection Alarm

- Identify a past relationship, belief, or experience that drains you and write out a mini cord-cutting letter.
- **Cord-Cutting Letter Structure**
  - What was the situation that created the trauma (who did it involve, how old were you, etc.)?
  - How did that make you feel emotionally?
  - If you could say anything to that person or people without repercussion, what would it be?
  - If you could say anything to yourself from back in that time, what would it be?
  - What did you learn from those experiences?
  - A line or two of forgiveness toward yourself.
  - A line or two of forgiveness toward others in the letter who hurt you.
  - After all is said and done, what are you the most grateful for in the aftermath of those situations?
  - A final sentence to close: "I clear any and all trauma, emotions, and contracts with the people and situations above, for the highest good of all involved."
  - Once it feels good, find a safe place to burn your letter, and journal about how it made you feel.

Observation Alarm

- Stop and observe the moment.
- Identify something in the moment that triggers you into a negative state.

- Observe your emotions around it without reaction.
- Document any observations you have around this process.

Pattern Disruptor

- Make a new and unexpected choice today.
- **Suggestion:** Do five random push-ups or jumping jacks.
- Write down what you chose and how your system responded to it.

WEEK 2: Navigate and Neutralize

Day 8: The Consumption vs. Creation Challenge

Reflection Alarm

- Set the intention to *create* more than you *consume* this week, and bring extra awareness to that balance.

Observation Alarm

- Stop what you're doing and observe the moment.
- Ask yourself if you are *consuming* or *creating* at this moment.
- Document what you observe in your notebook.

Pattern Disruptor

- Make a new and unexpected choice today.
- **Suggestion:** Take action on creating over consuming today. Write, draw, cook, record, build, or move your body.
- Write down what you did and anything else you noticed about it.

Day 9: Declutter One Space in Your Home

Reflection Alarm

- Look around you when this alarm goes off and ask yourself, **"What about this space makes me feel calm, or what about it makes me feel overwhelmed?"**
- Document your answer.

Observation Alarm

- Stop what you're doing and observe the moment.
- Ask yourself, **"Is the environment around me a current reflection of my mind?"**
- Document what you observe.

Pattern Disruptor

- Make a new and unexpected choice today.
- **Suggestion:** Pick one space (a drawer, your car, or your closet) and declutter it.
- Document the journey of clearing that space out. Did it make you feel overwhelmed at first? How did you feel after it was clean and organized?

Day 10: Identify Where Anxiety Comes From (Past, Present, Future)

Reflection Alarm

- Stop and reflect on where your anxiety has been coming from. Is it rooted in past wounds, stemming from present moment overwhelm, or focused on fears of the future?
- Document your reflections in your notebook.

Observation Alarm

- When the alarm goes off, stop and ask yourself these three questions:
    1. **"Is there anything from the past month that hasn't been resolved or is energetically lingering?"**
    2. **"Is there anything or anyone in the present moment that is negatively impacting me?"**
    3. **"Are there any fears I have about the future?"**
- Document these questions and answers in your notebook.

Pattern Disruptor

- Make a new and unexpected choice today.
- **Suggestion:** When you feel anxiety symptoms or notice an anxious thought today, refocus on your breath and your five senses.
- Write down what you did and any physical or emotional reactions you experienced during or after.

Day 11: Limit External Energy Drain

Reflection Alarm

- Reflect on the biggest energetic drain or area of overwhelm in your life.
- Document this reflection in your notebook.

Observation Alarm

- Stop and observe the moment.
- Ask yourself, **"What is my normal response during a moment of anxiety?"**
- Document what you observe in your notebook.

Pattern Disruptor

- Make a new and unexpected choice today.
- **Suggestion:** Put your phone on airplane mode for two hours.
- Document what you did differently in your notebook and how it felt.

Day 12: Choose Discomfort

Reflection Alarm

- Say this affirmation to yourself: **"I am safe even when I am uncomfortable."**
- Write it down, read it, and feel it deeply. Take a moment to visualize yourself being okay with discomfort.

Observation Alarm

- Stop and observe the moment.
- Ask yourself, **"What, if anything, makes me feel the most uncomfortable?"**
- Document what you observe in your notebook.

Pattern Disruptor

- Make a new and unexpected choice today.
- **Suggestion:** Take a cold shower, and observe the sensations and reactions both in your mind and body. You can switch from cold to hot and observe the difference in your reaction.
- Document this experiment in your notebook.

Day 13: Reprogram Anxiety

Reflection Alarm

- Reflect on any future fears or worries you may have and write them down in your notebook.

Observation Alarm

- Stop and observe the moment.
- Ask yourself, **"Is there anything I'm currently doing to control or micromanage a situation in order to prevent the worst-case scenario?"**
- Document what you observe in your notebook.

Pattern Disruptor

- Make a new and unexpected choice today.
- **Suggestion:** Take a moment to play a future anxiety scenario out in your head. Observe the reaction and symptoms in your mind and body. Remind yourself that you are safe and breathe if needed. Notice how it peaks, then fades. Review it over and over until it no longer holds an emotional reaction.
- Write down what Pattern Disruptor you tried today, and make note of any physical or emotional reactions you experienced during or after.

Day 14: Connected or Disconnected?

Reflection Alarm

- Say this affirmation to yourself: **"I am ready to take full responsibility over all aspects of my life."**
- Write it, read it, and feel it deeply.

Observation Alarm

- Stop and observe the moment.
- Ask yourself, **"What parts of this moment do I feel most present with or emotionally connected to?"** and **"What's happening around or within me right now that I am disconnected from?"**
- Document these interactions in your notebook.

Pattern Disruptor

- Make a new and unexpected choice today.
- **Suggestion:** Work on connecting and disconnecting from aspects of your day. Remember to utilize your five senses, cord-cutting techniques, and breath to direct your focus.
- Write down one thing you connected to and one thing you disconnected to and how you experienced them in your notebook.

WEEK 3: Utilize and Manifest

Day 15: Apply ReNU to an Anxious Moment

Reflection Alarm

- Say the affirmation to yourself: **"I am stronger than my anxiety."**
- Write it, read it, and feel it deeply. Take a moment to visualize yourself overcoming any anxious thought that arises.

Observation Alarm

- Stop and observe the moment.
- Ask yourself, **"How am I feeling energetically right now?"**
- Document what you observe in your notebook.

Pattern Disruptor

- Make a new and unexpected choice today.
- **Suggestion:** Ask yourself at this moment, **"Am I feeling anxious?"** If the answer is "yes," continue with applying the ReNU method:
    1. Recognize and ask: **"I feel anxiety—what is it trying to tell me?"**
    2. Neutralize and affirm: **"I am safe. I do not need to fear this feeling."**
    3. Utilize and ask: **"How can I use this moment for growth?"**
- Document this check-in in your notebook.

Day 16: Self-Love

Reflection Alarm

- Check in with yourself at this moment and ask, **"How are you doing? How is your body feeling? Where are your emotions at?"**
- Document this internal conversation in your notebook.

Observation Alarm

- Check in with yourself and ask, **"How are you feeling at this moment? Is there anything I can do to support you better?"**
- Document what you observe in your notebook; take action on giving back to yourself.

Pattern Disruptor

- Make a new and unexpected choice today.
- **Suggestion:** Do one thing today that is just for you. Maybe it's taking a bath, or watching your favorite movie, or sitting with the sunset. Give some extra love to yourself today, no matter how busy life gets. Put yourself first, even just for a moment.
- Document this self-love action in your notebook and how it made you feel.

Day 17: Shift Your Perspective

Reflection Alarm

- Say this affirmation to yourself and set an intention: **"I am ready to show up and shift my current state of being."**
- Write it, read it, and feel it deeply.

Observation Alarm

- Stop what you're doing and observe the moment.
- Focus on one aspect that is negatively impacting you right now. After bringing your awareness to it, shift your perception by finding something about it you can be grateful for.
- Document what you observe in your notebook.

Pattern Disruptor

- Make a new and unexpected choice today.
- **Suggestion:** Shift your autopilot response by doing something completely random: Clap loudly, throw a pen (safely) across the room, or laugh at an inappropriate moment. Making it extra uncomfortable is always a bonus.
- Document what you did differently and how both your body and mind responded.

Day 18: Manifest Something Small

Reflection Alarm

- Say this affirmation to yourself: **"I am a powerful manifester."**
- Write it, read it, and feel it deeply. Visualize yourself manifesting the life you've always dreamed of.

Observation Alarm

- Choose something small and completely random to manifest. It could be a cup of coffee, a sign from the universe, or an anxiety-free day.
- Write down what you want to manifest in your notebook. Remember that the more you focus on it, the faster it will come. Also remember that you need to picture yourself *already having* that thing.
- Be open to *how* it gets manifested, and document when it happens in your notebook.

Pattern Disruptor

- Make a new and unexpected choice today.
- **Suggestion:** Compliment someone out of the blue.
- Write down what you did and the interaction that played out after.

Day 19: Rewire Fear into Trust

Reflection Alarm

- Say this affirmation to yourself: **"I am ready to let go of control and trust in my higher contracts."**
- Write it in your notebook, read it, and feel it deeply.

Observation Alarm

- Stop what you're doing and observe the moment.
- Ask yourself, **"What about this moment am I not fully trusting?"**
- Document your observations in your notebook.

Pattern Disruptor

- Make a new and unexpected choice today.
- **Suggestion:** Find something to transmute. If there isn't one thing you can pinpoint today, then find something in your mind that negatively impacts you. Focus on it, and find one aspect of it that you can be grateful for.
- Write down what you transmuted and how you felt before and after the perception change.

Day 20: Embrace the Unknown

Reflection Alarm

- Say this affirmation to yourself: **"I have all the tools I need to embrace and navigate the unknown."**
- Write it, read it, and feel it deeply. Take a moment to visualize yourself facing something uncertain and being able to show up to it without fear.

Observation Alarm

- What were the more impactful reflections and Pattern Disruptors for you over the past twenty days? Go back and highlight or make a note of those in your notebook. When you have a moment of anxiety in the future, revisit these affirmations and activities.

Pattern Disruptor

- Make a new and unexpected choice today.
- **Suggestion:** Notice and question a spidey sense alert. Let your curiosity lead you into insights you weren't aware of before.
- Write down what you chose and how it affected you.

Day 21: Celebrate Your Transformation

Task: Write down three ways you've changed in the past twenty-one days.

- What feels different?
- How have I responded in different ways?
- What am I aware of now that I haven't been aware of before?
- What has improved?
- What can I continue to practice that has made the biggest impact?

Reflection Alarm

- Say this affirmation to yourself: **"I am strong enough to take on the uncertainty of the world, and navigate it with ease."**
- Write it, read it, and feel it deeply. Take a moment to visualize yourself anxiety free, with only gratitude, awareness, and calm in your mind.

Observation Alarm

- Stop what you're doing and observe the moment.
- Feel into your mind and body. Note any differences you have, compared to when you first observed this alarm twenty-one days ago.
- Document the differences in your notebook.

Pattern Disruptor

- Do one thing today to celebrate your journey. You have officially survived twenty-one days of awareness, action, and challenging your autopilot responses!

- Document what you did to celebrate in your notebook and how it feels to finish the twenty-one-day survival guide!

CONGRATULATIONS!

You did it! You've officially completed the twenty-one-day anxiety survival guide! This guide was designed to give you structure, confidence, and momentum as you integrate the powerful tools from this book into your daily life. Right now, you have everything you need to navigate the world with clarity, ease, and grace. Anxiety doesn't disappear overnight, and it's not about eliminating life's challenges. It's about being able to choose how and when you engage with the world around you. It's about freeing your mind from the constant mental noise. It's about feeling empowered to make choices that truly serve *you*, not everyone else. Just remember, true freedom from anxiety isn't a quick fix; it's a commitment to showing up for yourself every single day. The more you do, the calmer, clearer, and more in control you'll feel. And just because the twenty-one days are over doesn't mean your journey is. Keep applying what you've learned, and you'll gain the power to break free from anxiety, not just in the moment, but for life.

Acknowledgments

Writing a book about anxiety has been, ironically, both the most exhilarating and anxiety-inducing experience of my life. I could not have made it through this beautifully chaotic process without the extraordinary humans in my orbit who kept me grounded, inspired, and caffeinated.

First and foremost, an enormous thank-you to Glenn Yeffeth and the incredible team at BenBella Books for believing in this project from day one. A special shout-out to my brilliant editor, Claire Schulz. You lovingly whipped my chaotic downloads into clear, grounded brilliance (and somehow made it all make sense). Your patience and clarity were everything.

To my fierce literary dream team, Tessa Shaffer and Marissa Corvisiero, thank you for championing this book into existence with grace, grit, and relentless belief. You've both been cheerleaders through every twist and turn of this process, and I'm endlessly grateful.

To my luminous PR queen, Mona Loring, thank you for leading the charge in helping this message find the hearts that need it most. You are equal parts powerhouse and heart-healer, and this book is brighter because of you.

And, of course, to everyone in my life who has supported me through my own anxiety: the friends who answered late-night "Am I dying?" texts with memes, the family members who reminded me to breathe (and occasionally fed me), and the beings (both physical and otherworldly) who walked beside me through it all . . . thank you for showing me that healing is possible, that peace is real, and that love always wins.

This book is for the seekers, the feelers, the overthinkers, and the wildly courageous souls learning to come home to themselves. I see you. I love you.

And hey, if I can move through anxiety and come out the other side with a published book, you can absolutely do anything.

Anxiety Glossary

Anxiety Spiral: A mental loop where your mind repeatedly imagines negative or stressful scenarios, leaving you feeling trapped in worry and unable to escape.

Autopilot Programming: Refers to the subconscious belief systems, habits, and behaviors that operate without conscious awareness, often shaped by societal conditioning, past experiences, and ancestral influences.

Autopilot System: Your unconscious reaction pattern, where you mentally "check out" of certain experiences because they're familiar, unimportant, or overwhelming.

Chronic Anxiety: Persistent, long-term anxiety caused by suppressed emotions, unresolved past trauma, or ongoing emotional overwhelm.

Co-creation: The idea that you actively shape your life experiences and reality through your intentions, beliefs, and choices alongside other conscious beings and the universe.

Conscious Awareness: Fully present attention and intentional recognition of your current physical, emotional, and energetic state.

Conscious Connection: Deliberately engaging your attention and senses with something in your environment, physically or energetically.

Conscious Disconnection: Intentionally disengaging your emotional or physical attention from a situation, thought, or person to regain mental clarity.

Conscious Mind: The active, aware aspect of perception that processes thoughts, logic, and decision-making in real time.

Cord Cutting: The intentional practice of severing unhealthy or unwanted attachments to people, entities, past experiences, or timelines. It frees your energy body from draining connections, restores sovereignty, and allows for higher vibrational alignment with your soul's path.

Destiny/Contracts/Blueprints: A pre-agreed-upon set of experiences decided by your soul and spirit guides before coming to Earth.

Disassociation: When your conscious awareness disconnects from the present moment, either from your physical body, emotional state, or environment, usually as a protective mechanism.

Dis-ease: The imbalance that occurs when we fall out of alignment, allowing lower vibrations like fear, stress, or resistance to manifest physically, emotionally, or spiritually.

Electromagnetic Frequencies (EMFs): Vibrational energy waves that exist all around us, influencing both our physical and energetic bodies.

Empath: A highly sensitive individual who absorbs and feels the emotions, energies, and frequencies of others.

Energetic Cord: An invisible emotional or energetic link formed between you and objects, people, or experiences you interact with, influencing your thoughts and feelings.

Energetic Input: Information your body senses beyond your five physical senses, often felt as intuition or vibes.

Energy Body: The subtle, nonphysical layer of yourself that senses and processes energetic information from the environment before your physical brain becomes aware.

Energy/Vibrational/Frequency: The subtle energetic state or "vibe" you emit or resonate with, influenced by thoughts, emotions, and surroundings.

Extrasensory Abilities: The ability to tap in to energy or information that exists beyond the physical realm.

Fight, Flight, or Freeze Response: Your automatic survival reaction when feeling threatened, either fighting, fleeing, or becoming frozen and inactive.

Free Will: The divine ability to make choices independent of external control, karmic contracts, or programmed belief systems.

Hyperawareness: An intense sensitivity to subtle changes in your surroundings or emotions, often leading to anxiety.

Incarnation: The process by which a soul chooses to enter a physical body to explore set experiences in order to learn and grow.

Intuition: The direct knowing that transcends logic and reasoning, acting as a bridge between higher consciousness and the physical mind.

Metaphysical: Related to realities beyond physical matter and senses, including energetic and spiritual dimensions of experience.

Neural Pathways: Patterns in the brain formed by repeated thoughts, emotions, or behaviors, shaping automatic responses and habits.

Neutrality: The state of complete balance and nonattachment to polarizing energies. It's the ability to observe reality without judgment, fear, or emotional reactivity, allowing you to remain centered no matter what external chaos unfolds.

Objective Observation: Looking at a situation or thought without emotional judgment or reaction, enabling clarity and reducing anxiety.

Oversaturated Sponge Syndrome: Feeling overwhelmed due to absorbing too many emotions, energies, or external inputs, causing exhaustion and anxiety.

Reality: Not a fixed, objective experience but a fluid construct shaped by perception encompassing all that we see and more.

Solar Flares: Bursts of electromagnetic energy from the sun, believed to trigger energetic changes and upgrades in your brain and emotional sensitivity.

Soul: An eternal, energetic being of consciousness that exists beyond the physical body, experiencing many lifetimes to evolve, learn, and expand its awareness.

Spidey Sense: Your intuitive internal alarm system signaling that something is different or potentially unsafe, triggering anxiety.

Spirit Guides: Nonphysical beings, often souls who are highly evolved, ancestors, angels, or members of your spirit family, who assist, guide, protect, and support you throughout your life journey, helping you navigate challenges and align with your blueprints/contracts.

Subconscious Mind: The deeper, automatic part of your mind responsible for habitual reactions, memories, and emotional responses beneath conscious awareness.

Timeline: A potential path or trajectory of reality based on energy, choices, and frequency. Timelines are not fixed—they shift and change depending on individual and collective consciousness.

Transmutation: The conscious transformation of a negative or stressful emotional state into a positive or empowering one through mindful intention and awareness.

Vibrational Navigation (VN): Consciously choosing when and how deeply you connect or disconnect emotionally and energetically with your surroundings.

About the Author

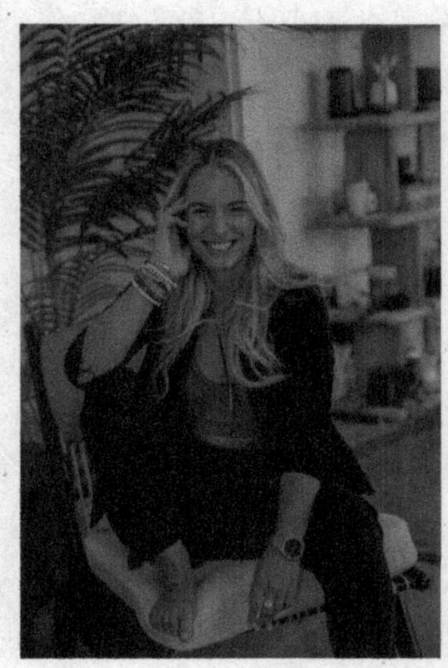

Elizabeth April is a spiritual coach and truth seeker who is deeply passionate about guiding humanity toward awakening. Known as EA, she is a bestselling author whose work has been featured by networks such as *Vice*, *Bustle*, Discovery, and Peacock. Elizabeth has shared her insights at conferences across North America. Her mission is to inspire positive global change and help unlock humanity's true potential. Are you ready to join her on this transformative journey?